MAKING THE VITAMIN CONNECTION

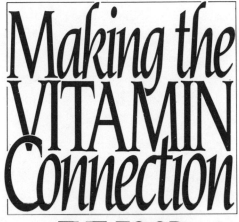

Making the VITAMIN Connection

THE FOOD SUPPLEMENT STORY

James Scala, Ph.D.

1817

HARPER & ROW, PUBLISHERS, New York

Cambridge, Philadelphia, San Francisco, London
Mexico City, São Paulo, Singapore, Sydney

FIRST EDITION

Designer: C. Linda Dingler

Library of Congress Cataloging in Publication Data

Scala, James.
  Making the vitamin connection.

  Bibliography: p.
  Includes index.
  1. Vitamins in human nutrition. 2. Dietary
supplements. 3. Minerals in human nutrition.
4. Vitamin therapy. I. Title.
QP771.S58   1985   613.2′8   85–42590
ISBN 0–06–015107–2

85 86 87 88 89 10 9 8 7 6 5 4 3 2 1

This book is dedicated to mothers.

Mothers have always been the true practitioners of nutrition. Their important influence begins at conception and continues after birth in shaping our entire relationship with food. And this relationship makes us what we are and what we become. The pages of this book attempt to explain how mothers managed to develop methods to supplement an ordinary diet long before the very nutrients involved were even understood. Even more marvelous are the means by which this information was preserved and passed on to other generations. Through the many ages these folk tales have supported us and allowed us not just to survive, but to thrive. And now we know that optimum health is within our grasp.

CONTENTS

Foreword

PAUL SALTMAN, PH.D.

Browse through any local bookstore or examine the paperback racks at the airport and you'll be overwhelmed by the number of titles that promise to bring you everlasting happiness, longer life, beautiful bodies, freedom from allergies, cures for diseases, and any state of mental or physical being you might desire. All you have to do is follow the author's special diet plan. So why, you might think, does the world need another book on nutrition?

Those who write about nutrition for the nonscientific public bear a great responsibility. Our country's Constitution guarantees anyone the right to say or print just about anything. The temptation to exploit people's ignorance and fears about their health by promising easy answers is great. Unfortunately, many self-appointed nutrition "experts" enrich themselves on the gullibility of others.

Why do we need books on nutrition? Human societies developed eating habits long before nutrition became a science. We only began to understand nutrition in the relatively recent past—the last century.

But long before the chemical isolation and characterization of nutrients, observation and religious beliefs attributed health-giving values to various foods and concoctions. Many of these dietary practices can now be justified and explained on the basis of nutritional studies. Eating burnt sea sponges prevents goiter because of their iodine content. The belief that apples pierced with nails help anemia can be substantiated by modern knowledge about iron. The old belief that garlic is good for the blood can be supported by experiments showing cholesterol-lowering and anti-coagulating effects of garlic extract. The healing reputation of certain waters that led to the establishment of many spas throughout the world stems from their trace mineral content. Thus there seems to be a historical precedent for adding substances to the diet, not to satisfy hunger but to safeguard health.

The modern scientific era for nutrition began with organic chemistry and the classification of nutrients in foods during the nineteenth century. The growth of knowledge accelerated with the identification of most vitamins from 1900 to 1948, followed by the subsequent discovery of trace elements such as iron and zinc. The establishment of human nutritional requirements and the nutrient analysis of foods have had an enormous impact on the health of our nation and the world.

An official U.S. government position on human nutritional requirements was first presented in the form of Recommended Dietary Allowances (RDA) tables during World War II, a time when America's food supply could not be taken for granted. Revised and updated about every four to six years, the RDAs occasionally lag behind new discoveries but still provide the most accurate overall reference of human nutritional needs at various ages.

Yet, in the midst of all this wonderful new knowledge rooted in tradition and folklore, something terrible has happened. Lulled by medical science's control of infectious disease, many people pay no attention to the nutritional aspects of their diets, leaving themselves vulnerable to marginal deficiencies and less than optimal health. As year of neglect follows year of neglect, dietary problems accumulate, ultimately cutting short or plaguing with illness the elderly years. There are, of course, people who are extremely concerned about their health. But they too know little if anything of modern nutrition science, and our ever mobile society, which erodes the community and extended family, has effectively cut off the flow of folklore and "old wives' tales" that once supplied nutrition advice.

Into this void step the charlatans and hucksters. They

choose to ignore the RDAs and clinical science. Their goal is to exploit people's ignorance and fear regarding their health. Shoving aside knowledge that has taken centuries to evolve, they promise overnight miracles in the form of untested magic pills and diets.

Alas, the bizarre regimens they advocate and the avalanche of overdoses—not one, not two, but often one hundred times the RDA—may cause more problems than they solve. The delicate balance of nutrients conducive to health can be disturbed not only by deficiencies but by vast excesses of individual nutrients, which can be toxic or interfere with the other essential nutrients.

That is why the world needs this book on nutrition. People need to get the story straight and Dr. Scala is the ideal person to do it. He has an impeccable scientific background stemming from his work as a research nutritionist during his graduate studies for the Ph.D. degree at Cornell University. He has published in scientific journals papers concerning fundamental aspects of nutrition science, foods, and food processing. He has worked in nutrition research as well as in the applied aspects of nutrition. Above all he has the ability to communicate valid scientific concepts with ease and charm to the average person.

This is the perfect book for both those who have never read anything on nutrition and those who are weary of fads and falsehoods. Through folk tales and nutrition lore, Dr. Scala gives us a perspective on nutritional practices that have stood the test of time and the tests of modern nutrition laboratories. In addition, he elaborates on some of the latest theories on nutrition and disease. By describing the methods our ancestors developed to meet their nutrient needs, setting forth the present-known roles and requirements for these nutrients, and explaining how they can best be obtained in contemporary society, Dr. Scala gives you the information you need to plan your meals and use supplements wisely.

Plus the reader is in for a treat. This book is delightful, delicious, and nutritious—a banquet for the mind.

PREFACE

Just as the universe is stranger than we can imagine, so is the human body more marvelous than we can fully realize. And with each new tool of research more of its secrets are uncovered, allowing us to marvel at its elegant simplicity.

Nutrition is the foundation of human health, which is built upon the genetic threads passed to us by our parents through the fabric of countless generations. It is a science that is evolving and developing with the tools of science and with the ever-changing human environment. These changing forces make this book, or any book on nutrition, a sort of Instamatic snapshot of human knowledge.

I know that some of the concepts in these pages will be proven less than complete, wide of the mark, or, in a word, "wrong," in view of findings being made at this instant or some-time in the future. Yet the basic principles are sound and will change very little. In fact, that is why history has played such a significant role in the story of supplementation, for it tells us how little some of our needs have changed. It should cause us to look back and realize just how abundant nature is and how marvelous are the tools that have allowed us to improve on it.

But, while the lessons of history bring to the fore the preventive role of nutrition, they also show us that abuses and excesses are wrong and, in some cases, criminal. Therefore, the reader should recognize that while supplementation is a tool for building health, supplements are not medicines that people can use at will on their own. Indeed, therapy is the domain of the science of medicine, and when nutrients are required in that domain, they need the guiding hand of the physician. That was true in the time of Hippocrates and it is still true today.

I want the reader to have respect for the nutrients. The idea that if a little is good more must be better is simply wrong. Any materials that can have such profound effects as to prevent night blindness or guard against deformation or reduce blood-platelet aggregation can be used to excess and cause serious health problems and even death. And, although some will say there is no upper limit for some nutrients, I would say our knowledge at present hasn't identified the upper limit, but it will.

With these principles and concerns in mind, the reader should enjoy this book. It tells of human inventiveness and how people developed some simple commonsense means to support their nutritional health.

JAMES SCALA

ACKNOWLEDGMENTS

Nutrition is too important to leave its communication to nutritionists. Without the creative hand of Deborah Prager, this book would not have been as interesting. Debbie converted my manuscript into prose that makes nutrition come alive. Debbie and I are indebted to Craig Comstock for final editing.

Dr. Gene Spiller, a friend, colleague, and scientist of international standing, examined the manuscript for technical accuracy. His fine scientific consideration and patience are appreciated. Gene was assisted by Carol Chuck, Carol Ikemiya, Chris Jensen, Les Wong, and Valerie Wookey to verify all factual information.

I owe a special debt of thanks to Chris Hollis for an outstanding job of manuscript production. Thanks are also due to Harriet Nicolay, Mabel Rich, and Linda Catala for the many drafts they typed.

As to my family, who lived this book at the dinner table, they deserve my thanks but, most of all, my apologies.

J.S.

I

FIBER

An Apple a Day

Everyone has heard that "an apple a day keeps the doctor away," but have you ever wondered what this old saying really means? Just why is that daily McIntosh or Granny Smith so good for your health?

It's not because of the apple's vitamin and mineral content. Apples contain some potassium, but only small amounts of other minerals and vitamins.

And it's not because the apple delivers many calories of energy. A medium-sized apple, say about a third of a pound (or 150 grams), yields about 90 calories. An equal weight of rib roast delivers some 660 calories, more than seven times as many. There's hardly any protein or fat in an apple, and you could get the carbohydrates from many other foods. What is special about an apple then? Bulk. In other words, fiber, the structural material that's found in all plants. Apples are an excellent source of dietary fiber.

Fiber is not a nutrient in the classic sense, the way protein or vitamins and minerals are. It's not absorbed into the bloodstream for delivery to cells and tissue. Quite the reverse: most fiber is not digested by our bodies. Most of it is just passing through—and it takes other waste materials along with it.

The "apple a day" aphorism must have originated in England, because only in English do the lines rhyme. Rosy-cheeked, healthy old farm folk were probably asked by the village doctor or their city cousins how they stayed so healthy. Imagine the farmer and his wife stopping and thinking for a minute. "Well," the farmer could have replied, "I eat an apple every day. We all do. Not a day goes by without my family and me eating apples."

It was fiber, sometimes called the body's broom, that kept the doctor away from these English folk and caused their reliance upon the apple to become immortalized in the proverb.

Fiber, the Forgotten Nutrient

The old English country folk couldn't have known all the specific ways in which fiber benefits health. Even now we're just beginning to recognize fiber's role. There's still no daily requirement established for fiber as there is for vitamins and minerals. That's why I call it "the forgotten nutrient."

In the last few decades, medical scientists have suggested that diseases common to affluent modern societies are due, in part, to a shift from diets high in fiber to those characterized by refined white flour and sugar. A decline in the consumption of foods high in fiber is now thought to play a role in the development of colon cancer, diverticular disease, obesity, varicose veins, hemorrhoids, gallstones, diabetes, and hiatus hernia. In addition, fiber has a special role in the elimination of toxic substances from the body.

Where Has All the Fiber Gone?

At the turn of the century, the average American ate about fifty-three pounds of apples a year. Today the average person eats about twenty pounds, which amounts to little more than one per week. Consumption of fiber, including whole grains, beans, fresh vegetables, and other fresh fruits, has dropped by 50 percent since 1910. What happened?

In 1870 the roller mill was invented. This machine enabled manufacturers to sell to the general public soft white flour that had heretofore been available only to the very rich. We can surmise that the introduction of white bread made from this flour as a replacement for stoneground wheat bread was the beginning of the end for fiber in the Western diet.

Industrialists soon found that processed foods had a longer shelf life, were tastier to the consumer, and could be mass manufactured and sold over a wide region. In some cases, processing removed fiber and inserted fats and sugars in its place.

In the ensuing decades, supermarket shelves were filling up with a panoply of increasingly altered versions of simple, whole grains, fruits, and vegetables. For example, you can now buy a "fruit" pie that contains no fruit pulp in the filling and no whole grains in the crust.

Ironically, a few aisles away from the fiber-depleted baked goods and convenience foods, you find shelves of laxatives to deal with constipation, caused, in large part, by the lack of fiber in today's overly processed diet.

Diseases of Affluence

As Americans started eating more fat and less fiber, more and more people began to become overweight. Heart disease skyrocketed to become the number one cause of death, with cancer close behind it.

At first nobody connected the emergence of these health problems to the removal of fiber from our diets. Fiber had been taken for granted. Through the ages it had always been a natural part of the food people grew for themselves, not only apples but wheat, oats, corn, millet, okra, chard, and beans.

By the twentieth century, however, the populace had migrated to the cities. Most people no longer lived on farms. They did not have access to fresh farm produce and were grateful for the convenience foods that industry had started to provide. As they became more affluent, they relied more and more on processed foods. But, with white bread instead of whole-wheat bread, large portions of meat instead of small portions mixed with beans, and mashed potatoes instead of whole potatoes, they were doing their health no favor.

The Fiber Revival

Much of the credit for shining the nutritional spotlight on fiber goes to Drs. Denis Burkitt and Hugh Trowell. These British medical missionaries spent about twenty-five years in Africa before returning to England in the early 1970s. In Africa they had noted the frequent passage of bulky stools and the low incidence of the diseases of affluence. They also noted that Africans consumed a diet high in vegetables and grains.

But what if dietary fiber wasn't the beneficial factor? What if there was something else, perhaps a genetic factor, that protected the Africans from diseases such as colon cancer and diverticulosis? To find out, scientists studied Africans who had moved to other parts of the world. They found that Africans who moved to industrialized nations and ate refined diets got these "Western" diseases as readily as non-Africans. The message seemed clear. Fiber is not mere waste. It's an important part of the diet.

When Burkitt and Trowell first published their work in the early 1970s, only a small group of health-food fans returned to the whole grains, fruits, and vegetables their parents had neglected. Today, however, United States government dietary guidelines urge all citizens to get enough fiber. Most people now realize that getting enough fiber a day is what helps keep the doctor away.

How Fiber Works

All foods that grow in fields or on trees and bushes contribute fiber—or what was once called "roughage"—to the diet. Foods of animal origin, meat and dairy products, do not. Nor do refined grain or certain types of fruit and vegetable products, because refining means the fiber has been removed. In the case of wheat, refining removes the bran. In fruits and vegetables, refining may remove the pulp. A dinner of macaroni and cheese with a bag of potato chips, washed down with a can of orange soda and followed by a dessert of ice cream and angel-food cake, would contain very little fiber. Yet this is the way many Americans now eat.

In digesting a meal, the body absorbs nearly all components, storing those not immediately needed as potential energy —perhaps more energy than the person can use, as we'll see soon. In contrast, fiber is not digested by our digestive enzymes. It's true that being chewed, fiber foods do release nutrients, various vitamins, and amino acids, depending on the food. But the bulk remains, and we now know that it has a vital physiological function.

One vital characteristic of fiber is its ability to bind water. Pectin, the kind of fiber in our daily apple, is especially good at this. As fiber moves through the body, it absorbs water, thus growing softer and larger. Think of the familiar form of fiber called a sponge. As it swells with water, a sponge becomes softer and binds other materials to its surface. That's how edible fiber works in the body, absorbing water and binding food residue. The result is a soft, bulky stool. This increases the frequency and ease of bowel movements. The most obvious benefits of sufficient fiber in the diet then are twofold: reduced "transit time" of all substances in the colon and elimination of straining. These benefits may have ramifications for human health. We will explore some of them in a moment.

Different Kinds of Fiber

As recently as ten years ago, scientists didn't really know how to measure fiber. They'd drop some into test tubes and slosh it around with acid and alkaline substances in an attempt to simulate human digestion. Then they'd filter the solution and measure what was left. What they didn't realize was that some forms of fiber dissolve in water. These include pectins, as in the apple and other fruits, and gums, as in oats and legumes. These are soluble fibers.

All that remained in the test tubes was a portion of the insoluble fibers—cellulose, hemicellulose, and lignin. These are the fibers found in most grains and vegetables. This portion came to be called "crude fiber." The sum total of all fibers is called "dietary fiber."

Today scientists' methods of fiber analysis are much more sophisticated. We've gone from measuring gross amounts of crude fiber to a more revealing analysis of fiber's action in the body.

Soluble and insoluble fibers work in different ways. The insoluble fibers such as the grains are the ones primarily responsible for increased moisture and bulk, which aid regularity. The soluble fibers, the pectins and gums, bind other digestive by-products, such as food residues and cholesterol, and help eliminate them.

Low-Fiber Diets and Overweight

Consider the volume of a head of cabbage and a small piece of chocolate that have approximately the same number of calories. You can chew and swallow the chocolate in the blink of an eye. And soon you'd probably want another piece. But twenty minutes may go by before you've eaten the entire head of cabbage. Chances are you won't be able to finish it—let alone want another one. That's why someone who eats a high-fiber diet rich in fruits and vegetables is not likely to be overweight.

It takes time to chew all those vegetables, beans, fruits, and cereals, whereas a diet devoid of fiber can be consumed very quickly. Since it takes about twenty minutes for the stomach to let the brain know that it's full, a person feasting on refined or fatty foods can drastically overeat before the brain can put a stop to it. In contrast, a person eating fibrous foods will put the fork down after consuming far fewer calories.

In weight control, calories are the name of the game. The amount of energy that foods provide and the amount of energy that a person burns through his or her basal metabolism plus daily activities are measured in calories. If you take in more calories than you burn, you develop an energy surplus in the form of excess body fat. To get rid of that fat you have to reverse the equation and, for a while, consume fewer calories than your body burns.

Because fiber is not digested it does not provide any calories to humans. To cows and some other animals, yes—they have the enzymes to break fiber down. Another bonus of fiber-rich fruits and vegetables is that they're 85 to 95 percent calorie-free water. But most people don't take advantage of low-calorie, high-fiber foods when trying to lose weight.

A Radical Change of Diet

Since prehistoric times, humans have tended to eat just over a pound (about 500 grams) of dry weight of food per day. Although fiber intake has decreased in our society, we still eat roughly the same amount of food per day. We're just eating different kinds of food. Affluence and technology allow us to develop and indulge a taste for fatty, sweet, and salty foods. But don't take my word for it. Go to a vending machine, a fast-food restaurant, and a convenience store, and compare the number of food choices containing fiber to those providing fat, sugar, and salt. Look at the contents of people's shopping carts when you're in line at the supermarket. How does the amount of fruit, vegetables, and grains being purchased stack up against the packages of meat, cookies, soda, snacks, crackers, cheese, pastries, and ice cream?

Not surprisingly, overweight has become our society's biggest health problem, affecting both children and adults. One of every four women and almost one of every five men in their forties are at least 20 percent above desirable weight. What's more insidious is that almost 40 percent of women above age forty are 10 percent or more overweight and over 30 percent of men in the same age group are more than 10 percent overweight. A person who is 20 percent over ideal body weight is medically considered obese and is at greater risk of dying of heart disease. Heart disease, as we stated earlier, is now the leading cause of death in our nation. Excessive weight is also a risk factor in cancer and stroke, the second and third most common causes of death respectively.

Part of the blame for this surely rests on our replacing a fiber-rich diet with calorie-dense processed foods and meats. The numbers speak for themselves. If we look at U.S. Army induction records, we see that in 1863 the average weight of a Civil War soldier, 5 feet 8 inches, 30 to 34 years old, was 147 pounds. Now remember the roller mill was invented in 1870. By 1965, his great-great-grandson weighed 165 pounds—nearly 20 pounds more than his Civil War ancestor!

Unfortunately, this trend shows no signs of abating. New government statistics show that children one year of age today are 50 percent heavier than children of the same age just a generation ago.

Economic and political factors make direct comparisons difficult between our society and many of those that subsist on high-fiber diets, such as the Asian and African nations. Instead, let us look at one Asian nation that has become prosperous, Japan. As average family income increased in this newly affluent nation, so did weight. As the traditional diet of rice, vegetables, and fish gives way to burgers, fries, and colas, the Japanese find they've imported another product of Western culture—overweight and the health problems that come along with it. For the first time ever, Japan has become a market for weight-control programs. A similar phenomenon can be noted among other Asian peoples who immigrate to the United States. Those who stick to their native diets tend to remain slim while those who adapt to Western cuisine start to put on pounds.

Fiber, in moderation, fills you up without filling you out. Take away fiber and what you've got left is calories and plenty of them, including sugars and fats. Fiber is nature's original diet food.

High-Fiber Foods and Cholesterol

One kind of fat that's become notorious as an artery clogger is cholesterol. And with good reason. High levels of cholesterol in the blood can line the walls of arteries and interfere with blood circulation in a condition known as atherosclerosis. If an artery becomes so clogged that blood can no longer get through, a heart attack occurs.

An apple a day and other sources of soluble fiber may have a role in preventing cholesterol buildup. The pectins and gums in fruits, oats, and beans seem to act as bouncers in the body. If a customer in a nightclub or bar becomes drunk and unruly a professional bouncer will firmly escort him to the door. Excess cholesterol is an unwelcome presence in the body's vital circulatory system. Pectins and gums, experiments show, bind cholesterol and substances that are produced by cholesterol and literally escort the excess to the body's exit. Experiments with intake of oat bran (different from wheat bran) and beans showed declines of up to 20 percent in blood-cholesterol levels.

Also, a diet high in fiber will usually be low in fat, and evidence shows that a low-fat diet aids in maintaining low blood-cholesterol levels and preventing heart disease. For the majority of the world's people who live on grains and vegetables, heart disease does not exist. They have other problems to be sure, but not heart disease. In our own society, studies on vegetarian population groups such as the Seventh Day Adventists reveal that they have lower cholesterol levels and less heart disease than Americans who eat diets high in animal fat.

Low-Fiber Diets and Cancer

When the U.S. government recently launched its first official nationwide cancer-prevention campaign, high on its list of recommendations was the advice to eat less fat and more high fiber foods, such as whole grains, beans, vegetables, and fruits.

Conclusive studies link high intake of animal fat to cancer, especially cancer of the breast and colon. Again, groups such as the Seventh Day Adventists who eat high-fiber and low-fat diets have lower rates of colon cancer than those who do the reverse. And a study found that women hospitalized for breast cancer were more likely to be constipated—the telltale sign of a diet lacking in sufficient fiber—than women hospitalized for other reasons.

What's the story behind the low-fiber diet-cancer connection? Again, it's partly the seesaw relationship between fiber and fat in the diet.

Since high-fiber foods are filling, eating more of them leaves less room for fattier foods. But there's more to it than that.

A diet high in fiber not only discourages excess intake of fats; it may help the body deal with toxic substances. Each kind of fiber plays its own role. Just as the soluble fibers—the pectins and gums—bind cholesterol and "escort" some of it out of the body, so they may also bind some toxic substances. On the other hand, the insoluble fibers—the cellulose, hemicellulose, and lignin found in vegetables and grains—increase fecal bulk and thus shorten the amount of time food stays in the colon. This may reduce the opportunity for potentially harmful substances to do any damage. The sluggish movement of solid waste through the body, such as occurs on a low-fiber diet, allows more time for any potential carcinogens present in the colon to possibly initiate cancer (see Chapter 13).

For example, let's say two people ingest the same amount of toxic material. One person eats a low-fiber diet and has a bowel movement every other day. The second person eats a high-fiber diet and has a daily bowel movement. The harmful substance would be in the former person's system twice as long. Over a lifetime, the cumulative effect could have quite serious consequences.

An experiment that supports these theories tested the effects of fiber in carcinogenic diets in animals. When a group of rats were fed a pure food diet, they developed healthy coats of fur and grew to normal size. When red dye No. 2, a carcinogen, was added, growth ceased, the fur thinned, and the rats died within two weeks. When a similar group were fed the same dye-laced diet mixed with fiber, the carcinogen effect was neutralized. All of the animals survived and grew to their full weight. The scientist concluded that the protective effect of the fiber was greater than could be accounted for by bulk alone. We can speculate that it was a combination of the properties of soluble and insoluble fiber that offered the animals some defenses against cancer.

Many high-fiber fruits and vegetables also contain beta-carotene, a nutrient we'll discuss in Chapter 13.

Low-Fiber Diets and Diabetes

Another disease closely linked with obesity is diabetes. Fiber seems to offer benefits here, too. Animal studies show that replacing a high-fiber diet with one rich in fat and sugar increases the risk of diabetes. Also, we know that diabetes is rare in societies in which fiber is a prominent part of the diet.

It's fiber's familiar bulk and spongelike properties that help to moderate the absorption of sugar into the bloodstream. Here is a simple experiment: Feed someone a large apple, and thirty minutes later he or she will still feel pleasantly full. Break up the cell walls by grinding that apple into sauce before offering it, and the person will feel less full. Run that apple through an apple press and filter out all the fiber, and you'll be left with the concentrated sweet liquid we call apple juice. After drinking the juice of one apple, your subject wouldn't feel the least bit satisfied.

But look what happens in each case to the subject's blood sugar! The sugar in the apple is absorbed very slowly, with a moderate insulin rise. The sugar in the applesauce is absorbed more quickly. The sugar in the apple juice hits the body the fastest, with the sharpest insulin response.

What makes the difference? The fiber in the apple, that's what. The sugar in the apple is suspended in a matrix of fiber. This slows the sugar's movement across the intestinal wall. When the sugar zooms across the intestinal wall quickly, as in the case of the apple juice, the pancreas gets a signal that says: "Big sugar has arrived. Release lots of insulin!" In many cases, the body's insulin production is likely to overshoot its mark. Excess insulin causes blood sugar to drop below what it was before the subject drank the apple juice. The person may feel irritable, hungry, and then tired. In the case of the apple, less sugar enters the system initially, calling forth a more appropriate amount of insulin and thus allowing blood sugar to stay more constant.

In some cases, high-starch, high-fiber diets have been

used effectively by physicians to help reduce the insulin medication of diabetics who required only low doses of insulin. Other studies have shown that the blood-sugar levels of patients taking insulin were significantly higher on a low-fiber diet than on a high-fiber diet. Of course, diabetics should not alter their diets without the advice of their physician.

Low-Fiber Diets, Diverticular Disease, and Hemorrhoids

A diet lacking in fiber produces hard stools rather than bulky soft ones, thus causing the body to strain in its efforts to excrete solid waste. The straining may be the leading factor in diverticular disease, hemorrhoids and, perhaps, as some scientists suggest, varicose veins.

When there is little bulk in the diet, pressure can build up in the intestine to help move solid waste along the intestinal tract. After years of a low-fiber diet, the intestinal surface may become irregular from the high pressure. This creates additional pressures and cramps, which then cause little pockets to bulge out in weakened areas of the intestinal wall. This is diverticular disease.

Virtually nonexistent in the early part of the twentieth century, diverticular disease has grown steadily in industrialized countries. Now an estimated one-fourth to one-third of the middle-aged and older people in Western nations have this condition. Yet the incidence of diverticular disease has changed little in populations such as the Chinese and the Africans whose traditional lifestyles protect them from modern food-processing technology. But when Asian and African people switch from their high-fiber diets to our "affluent" low-fiber diets, they too develop diverticular disease.

Laboratory studies also offer evidence of fiber's role in diverticular disease. Rats fed a fiber-free diet develop diverticulosis while those fed a fibrous diet do not.

When a person strains to eliminate solid wastes, pressure

is put on the entire abdominal region. This downward pressure works against the veins in the legs, which are carrying blood back to the heart. When these weakened veins burst, the result is the visible, maplike network of gray and purple lines we call varicose veins.

Likewise, straining can weaken blood vessels in the anus, causing them to become distended—a condition we call hemorrhoids. Hippocrates, the father of modern medicine, was one of the first to recognize hemorrhoids, which he attributed to dietary flaws. Modern science has confirmed his observations: hemorrhoids are associated with a low-fiber diet.

Lack of fiber and the resulting straining and constipation are also thought to play a role in appendicitis, gall bladder disease, and hiatus hernia. Although a lack of fiber may not cause these conditions, it probably promotes their development.

Getting Enough Fiber

In the old English farmer's diet, the daily apple rounded out his hefty daily intake of fiber. We fiber-depleted creatures of the twentieth century need to put back into our diets more fiber than an apple a day can provide, although it's not a bad way to start.

How can we work more fiber into our busy schedules? Business people and teens eat many meals out, and restaurants rarely provide much fiber. The two-career couple don't have the time to wash, peel, and cut all those vegetables and cook all those grains. The single person recoils at the thought of having to throw out all the sodden rotting produce that he or she didn't get around to finishing.

It may be impractical for some of us to follow a vegetarian diet, but it's simple to add quick forms of fiber to snacks and meals. Remember, you need more than one kind, so in addition to that apple be sure to sprinkle some unprocessed bran on your foods or snack on some fresh vegetables—or add a palatable fiber supplement that contains all the necessary forms of fiber.

You can opt for a fiber supplement and choose to learn to cook with old-fashioned grains, beans, and produce—but don't procrastinate. The health problems brought on by lack of fiber in the diet build up over the years and tend to strike in old age when we're most vulnerable. The sad thing is that so many of these problems could be avoided entirely or lessened. So get into the fiber habit and enjoy the many benefits it offers.

Introduction to the Fat-Soluble Vitamins

GENE SPILLER, PH.D.

The vitamins, the complex organic molecules found in our food that are essential to life, were long ago subdivided into two broad classes: the fat- (or oil-) soluble A, D, E, and K and the water-soluble B complex and C. While all the vitamins are essential to good health, it seems as though nature has made special provisions for the fat-soluble vitamins by enabling the human body to store them for much longer periods of time than the water-soluble vitamins. Vitamin D, for instance, is produced by the action of sunlight on the skin and, when sunlight is in short supply as in a northern winter, the vitamin can be stored by the body for a long time to prevent deficiencies.

These are the vitamins that prevent blindness and make good vision possible, ensure growth, and help build resistance to infections (vitamin A); they are the vitamins that ensure calcium absorption (vitamin D); that ensure blood coagulation after injury (vitamin K); and that help fight harmful by-products of metabolism (vitamin E).

Although fat-soluble vitamins are so carefully stored by the body, deficiencies do exist! For instance, vitamin A deficiency is rampant in poor countries. Millions of children become blind and some of them die.

Because vitamins A, D, and K are so well stored and their elimination is slow, they should never be consumed in excessive amounts. Vitamin E differs somewhat, as it has such

a grinding task day in and day out in our bodies: the task
of protecting cells from destructive by-products of various
metabolic reactions. Because of this ubiquitous role, vitamin
E can be consumed in amounts slightly higher than the
recommended intakes and still be safe.

In the last few years, in addition to the classic oil-
soluble vitamins (A, D, E, and K), beta-carotene, once
thought to be just a precursor of vitamin A, has created a
tremendous amount of interest for its possible protective
effect in some types of cancers.

Before you read the intriguing stories about each
of the vitamins in the chapters that follow, I will briefly
summarize their functions. Vitamins A and E are involved in
the protection of cells and tissues; additional functions of A
are to ensure vision and proper growth. The role of D is to
assist in calcium absorption and thus bone formation and
maintenance, and the role of K is to prevent excessive
bleeding and to quickly plug a damaged blood vessel. In
an even more general way, we can look at the fat-soluble
vitamins as the sentinels of proper growth and maintenance
of the integrity of our body structure, helping us fight
infection and protecting our precious trillions of body cells
from harm.

2

VITAMIN A

A Carrot for Alcor

In the handle of the Big Dipper, in the middle, are two closely associated stars, a bright one called Mizar and a very dim one known as Alcor. Long ago in the age of campfires and oil lamps, when the sky over cities was not yet shrouded in electric haze, the Arabs used Alcor as a test of good eyesight. If someone failed the test, they prescribed vegetables, most likely alfalfa, as a remedy.

Some 2,400 years ago, Hippocrates was aware of this test of night visual acuity. Like the Arab physicians before him, he sought to improve night vision by supplementing the diet, thus following his maxim "Let food be thy medicine." But, instead of using only vegetables, he prescribed liver—calf liver for those who could barely see Alcor or could see it only part of the time, beef liver for those who could not see the dim star at all. Although he didn't know what the therapeutic factor was, he realized that more of it was present in old animals than in young ones. This is characteristic of what we call a fat-soluble vitamin, in this case vitamin A.

In Biblical times fishermen knew that if their night vision, critical to their livelihood, had diminished, they could restore it in one day by simply eating the liver of a fish or a seagull. The ancient Chinese also recognized the value of fish and still use shark fin soup to supplement their diet. It's interesting that, like Hippocrates, they all recognized the efficacy of a food supplement that, like the Arabs' alfalfa or fish liver, was delivering vitamin A.

Enter the Carrot

In European folklore the benefits of vitamin A, such as its effect on night visual acuity, have, in the main, been associated with the carrot. The carrot is a member of the parsley family, which includes celery and parsnips. It evolved from the plant we know as Queen Anne's lace. Long recognized as a medicinal, the carrot has for centuries been a staple in soups and stews and, more recently, in salads. It contains a substance called beta-carotene, also found in sweet potatoes and leafy vegetables. In plants, beta-carotene is thought to help trap light for photosynthesis. It is also the precursor of vitamin A. Ingested by humans, beta-carotene is converted into vitamin A in the intestinal wall and in the liver. Thus, unlike many other vitamins, A is an animal product, although its precursor comes from plants.

  Vitamins have been discovered when a dietary substance was found to alleviate a disease symptom or restore a bodily function. People often originally assumed the disease was caused by germs. In the case of vitamin A, however, the first sign of deficiency was the loss of nighttime visual acuity, a condition long ago linked to nutrition. Thus, it is probably the first factor actually discovered as missing from a diet.

Vitamin A and Tissue Development

Vitamin A is required for cell differentiation, the process by which a proto-cell specializes and takes on a particular shape and set of complex functions. An especially important role is played by A in the smooth-surface tissues of the body, including the skin, the mucous membranes, the mouth, the eyes, the nose, and the entire digestive system. The human body has trillions of cells, most of which are continually being replaced. Each one depends on vitamin A to help it develop into what it's supposed to be, a knee cell, a throat cell, or whatever.

  Consider for example the skin, which is the body's largest

organ and covers the entire surface. A skin cell is formed well below the surface. As it migrates upward it typically changes from a round basal cell to a flattened cell when it reaches the surface. It also specializes, depending upon its location. In the nose, the mouth, the stomach, and the large intestine, it becomes a particular kind of mucous membrane. On the face, chest, or arm it differentiates into external skin. The process of differentiation requires vitamin A.

In the eye the basal cells differentiate into highly specialized surface cells. In the cornea of the eye, for example, the cells must be transparent. To the extent that they are clouded it's as if a camera had a dark filter on it or even a lens cap. Visual impairment or blindness occurs when cells in the eye tissue become keratinized, that is, amorphous, dry, and scaly. If you think of a corn or a callus on the toe and imagine eye tissue becoming like this you will have an idea of what it would be like to be blinded in this way. In some Third World countries where food is scarce, it's estimated that over 200,000 children become permanently blind each year because of lack of vitamin A. When martyrs go on starvation diets, as did imprisoned members of the Irish Republican Army in recent times, one of the symptoms reported by the media is the onset of night blindness, then total blindness.

Hair and fingernails are composed principally of keratin. But in most other tissue the growth of keratin is devastating. In the life of the large intestine, for example, it's the integrity of the walls that helps to prevent infections and toxic substances from entering the blood. A prolonged severe deficiency of vitamin A leads to keratinization of the delicate tissues and cracking of the walls. Cracking of this type can develop in many parts of the alimentary tract from the lips to the anus. Diarrhea begins and the body becomes less able to process food efficiently. Nutrients fail to be absorbed and infection sets in. As the deficiency progresses, external skin lesions may develop along with cracks, peels, and blisters. Eventually, death is the result.

Vitamin A and Mucus Production

Sensitive tissues such as lungs, intestine, and the mouth rely upon
the secretion of mucus to protect them and to help them perform
their special functions. Mucus is the body's lubricant; it helps
keep substances moving throughout the digestive system. When
vitamin A is deficient, mucus production may stop, the tissue
may crack and infection may begin. If vitamin A is then provided, the tissue barriers to infection can be restored. For this
reason, vitamin A has earned the name "the infection fighter" as
though it had some kind of antibiotic property. In fact, however,
vitamin A acts not by killing germs but by excluding them from
vulnerable tissues. Without mucus, certain tissues crack; with it
they remain strong and effective as a barrier against infectious
agents such as bacteria.

High Beta-Carotene Foods and Cancer

People once ascribed certain deaths to a disease they called "the
wasting disease." Today we know it as cancer. A myriad of factors
are involved in its development. Vitamin A may have a role to
play.

Think of a person living in a seacoast village in Japan or
in a reasonably prosperous part of rural Africa—a person who eats
unprocessed vegetables, fruits, and cereals more regularly than we
do and whose protein consists mainly of fish and poultry rather
than steaks or chops. Now imagine that this person's brother
immigrates to the U.S. or to Western Europe, where the air is
heavy with factory fumes, auto exhaust, and cigarette smoke, and
where the diet is much higher in fats and sugar at the expense
of vegetables. The man residing in the modern world has ten to
fifteen times as high a risk of developing cancer as his sibling back
home.

Many factors are involved in the development of cancer.
There is no one direct "cause," but the risk of cancer may be
increased by not eating fresh fruits and vegetables. In addition

to fiber, carrots and other fruits and vegetables provide many dietary factors, among them beta-carotene, which are somewhat low in the American diet. Now, nobody would claim that cancer is caused by the absence of carrots, red cabbage, sweet potatoes, green leafy vegetables, or liver, much less that it can be cured by eating these foods or by taking Vitamin A capsules. Consider, however, Dr. Richard Shekelle's studies on heavy smokers. One group had a diet typical of the U.S., while the other group had a more vegetarian diet rich in beta-carotene and in fiber (the subject of Chapter 1). Although the second group, consuming a diet rich in beta-carotene and fiber, had a higher rate of cancer than the average population of nonsmokers, this rate was substantially below that of their fellow heavy smokers who were eating a typical U.S. diet with its fat and sugar. The dietary factor that might have counted was beta-carotene, the precursor of vitamin A.

In recent years, scientists have developed some interesting theories on beta-carotene. One theory, proposed by Dr. Richard Peto, is that beta-carotene acts as an antioxidant in the body (a subject discussed in Chapter 4). A number of factors, including cigarette smoke and exhaust smoke as well as normal cell metabolism, produce substances called "free radicals" that are able to damage cells and may even lead to cancer. These free radicals and some other carcinogenic agents may be rendered harmless by beta-carotene.

More About Beta-Carotene

Beta-carotene comes in fruits and vegetables—it's what gives carrots, yams, pumpkins, and oranges their orange color. It is fat-soluble and stored in fatty tissue throughout the body, including the fat stores just under the skin. In fact, if you were regularly to drink a large amount of fresh carrot juice, certain parts of your skin would turn a slightly orange color. When the body needs vitamin A it simply converts some of this beta-carotene to the vitamin. As long as beta-carotene is available, the body can make as much vitamin A as it requires. However, the body does not have a means to excrete excess levels of preformed vitamin A, which are ingested directly in the form of fish-liver oil or animal liver or in food supplements. Thus large quantities of vitamin A can be toxic, while as of this writing large amounts of beta-carotene have proven safe.

The Vitamin A and Acne Myth

Acne is a problem for many teenagers and young adults. Anything that promises to help cure it has been pursued at great length, and vitamin A is no exception. Unfortunately, vitamin A in supplement form does not cure acne. The anti-infection properties of this vitamin were once thought to help acne, but research has found this not to be true. Recent studies have shown that topical and oral use of retinoic acid, a modified form of vitamin A, may interfere with the blemish-causing production of oil by sebaceous glands. However, the effect of this natural metabolite on acne is very limited and the amount required could have toxic effects; it should be administered only by a physician.

Isotretinoin, a drug chemically known as 13-cis-retinoic acid, has been found effective. It must be administered by a physician, usually a dermatologist, who is skilled in its use. It has some temporary side effects, such as giving the skin a rough, flaky texture, which is rather pronounced but disappears after the course of therapy. Nevertheless, it does require very serious and careful medical supervision. Also, Isotretinoin should not be used by pregnant women.

There is one other connection between vitamin A and acne that should be discussed. For vitamin A to be activated, zinc is required. Studies with zinc and acne have yielded some results with some teenagers. At first it was thought that zinc was effective because it helped the body to mobilize its vitamin A. As more research was done, Dr. Gerd Michaëlsson found that zinc's beneficial effect on some teenage acne may have been the result of the zinc itself. Consequently, vitamin A doesn't appear to have a significant effect on the clearing up of acne. However, curiosity about vitamin A led to therapeutically useful discoveries about retinoic acid.

Who Needs Vitamin A?

In today's world two broad classes of people are not obtaining sufficient beta-carotene and vitamin A foods. One is the impoverished people who do not have the opportunity to get the right kinds of foods and obtain the necessary nutrients. Severe deficiency accounts for about 25,000 deaths per year.

The other class of people who are affected, although more subtly or indirectly, by this type of dietary inadequacy are among the richest in the world, living in economically developed countries. A recent survey showed that 30 percent of Americans get insufficient vitamin A, probably because of lack of vegetables and seasonal fruits. Americans have come to favor processed foods loaded with fat and sugar and muscle meat rather than organ meat, which is rich in vitamin A.

Even if we get enough beta-carotene to preserve our night vision and to facilitate cell differentiation—enough to meet the government's criteria of satisfactory health—we still may not be ingesting sufficient quantities. Given the toxicity of auto exhaust, factory fumes, and power-plant emissions, I believe there is really no one in the cities of the U.S. who doesn't "smoke." Dr. Shekelle has shown that the consumption of beta-carotene-containing foods somewhat reduced the risk of lung cancer in smokers and nonsmokers (however, it should be emphasized that cigarette smoking increases the risk of other serious diseases and there is no evidence that dietary carotene affects these other risks in any way). It is, of course, wise to avoid smoking and inhaling "secondhand" smoke and other pollutants. To the degree that modern life requires antioxidant protection against these oxidative pollutants and carcinogens, I believe that beta-carotene should be considered not simply a vitamin A precursor but as a nutrient in its own right with its own antioxidant properties. In addition to the question of how much vitamin A we need as a recommended dietary allowance we should also ask how much beta-carotene the body needs, not only to produce vitamin A but to perform additional antioxidant functions.

Toxicity of Excessive Vitamin A

Excessive vitamin A, such as 50,000 IU per day taken regularly for months, can cause serious medical problems. Sometimes even lower amounts may cause problems. The greatest danger is to infants and children, although adults can experience toxicity. In all age groups, a major excess of vitamin A can actually cause death. One polar expedition became seriously disabled after eating bear liver. It seems the polar bear eats so much fish and its liver is so large that it contains enough vitamin A actually to poison people. At all ages excessive vitamin A can cause joint pain, rash, itchiness, enlarged liver, loss of appetite, and, in women, cessation of menstruation. The symptoms disappear very quickly when the vitamin A intake stops. In contrast, an elevated level of beta-carotene may produce a slightly yellow skin but it does not produce vitamin A toxicity.

Supplementation

A carrot can serve not only as homage to Alcor but, perhaps, as a kind of filter for the air we have no choice but to inhale. However, not everyone in modern society walks around with a briefcase of carrot sticks or a slice of red cabbage. To keep up with our busy schedules we resort to fast foods such as hamburgers, and when we relax we have come to prefer highly processed "gourmet" foods, which may offer more chic than nutritional balance. It's a question how many people can bring themselves to carry a small bag of carrot sticks with them to work each day or make sure that they've eaten a sufficient portion of red cabbage, brussels sprouts, squash, or the like.

In societies of old, meat was sufficiently scarce so that it was sort of a supplement to help improve the quality of the protein in other foods and to add flavor. Our society has exactly reversed the process: the vegetable has become the condiment. We have cut down considerably on our consumption of seasonal vegetables and fruits. At best we have made salads into a side dish. Nowadays carrots are likely to be mere shreds on top of a salad.

To some extent, we have separated the sensual pleasure of eating from the healthful necessities of nutrition. We prefer the flavors of meats, pastries, and salted snacks to those of fresh vegetables and fruits. While the food engineers provide a plethora of food pleasures, it is left to nutritionists to supplement the diet with vitamins, minerals, and other factors our bodies need. Now, fortunately, the same engineering techniques that allow food to be processed can also make available supplements that are both portable and palatable.

Beta-carotene should be regarded both as a known nutrient and, beyond that, perhaps, as a form of insurance policy against factors that may contribute to health problems. As in the case of vitamin C, there is little evidence that beta-carotene, in reasonable amounts, causes any problem and substantial evidence to suggest that it can help to assure optimum health. Eat a carrot for Alcor and, if that's inconvenient, take a beta-carotene supplement.

3

VITAMIN D

Sun Worship

In the thirteenth century the little city of Weistar, in what is now East Germany, had streets so narrow that most windows admitted very little direct sunlight. The streets were wide enough for a horse-drawn cart but not wide enough to allow the sun to reach the windows, except when it was nearly overhead. In the winter, therefore, the residents had little access to sunlight except on their faces and hands when they went out-of-doors. In any case the winter sun in that part of the world is too low in the sky to be of much value. When the sun is at an oblique angle, ultraviolet light is more severely attenuated by the atmosphere. Therefore, not only was the end of winter a time for planting crops, it was also the time when people in northern cities could receive ample sunshine, hence ample vitamin D. Sun worship must have had some roots in the human body's need for the sunshine vitamin.

The women in Weistar and in most parts of the northern world had a saying that every child must get the January sun. In the coldest part of winter, a mother had to carry her child to a park and disrobe the child as much as possible to get the sun. Adults got enough sun in the course of their daily activities, but over the years mothers had noticed that babies born in the fall had a lower rate of survival than babies born in the spring and that among winter children who survived there was a higher rate of deformities. At first people thought the cause might be the cold or the winter diet, but folk wisdom said it was the scarcity of sunlight. Thus, the older women would tell the mothers of winter babies to watch for a day without too much wind when the temperature was warm for the season and then let those little bodies soak up the sun.

When historians examined the Weistar church records, they indeed found that a child born in the late fall had the lowest chance of survival. Inscriptions on gravestones showed that more children died in the winter than in the spring. Clearly, having been conceived around the Maypole was a disadvantage because it meant being born in the white months when the sun was low and people stayed indoors. In contrast, the autumn baby could store enough vitamin D in the liver to get through the winter. The winter baby would be faced with not getting enough vitamin D during the most important growth period and deformities would result. Unless enough vitamin D was provided from mother's milk, the child absolutely needed the January sun.

Industrial Society

In nineteenth-century England during the Industrial Revolution, smoke and buildings darkened the skies of the cities. Unable to get adequate sunlight, many children developed bowlegs and poorly-formed arms, hands, and feet. Tiny Tim, the character created by Charles Dickens, may have been a product of these conditions.

Take a third example—Detroit from 1910 to 1920. During this period, which preceded the Great Depression and was part of America's industrial expansion, 20 percent of schoolchildren showed evidence of at least minor bone deformity, a disease that has become known as rickets (you've heard someone call a warped structure "rickety"). In Detroit, as in Weistar or Manchester, England, the winter sun is low in the sky. The automobile had been invented and smoke from the new factories suddenly shrouded whatever sun had slanted down. Many children were forced to work in places where even the remaining sunlight could not reach. Consequently, vitamin D deficiency was a major problem.

During the 1920s and 1930s while children in Detroit and other northern industrial centers were suffering from rickets, the science of nutrition was showing the necessity of supplementing the diet with vitamin D.

The first idea was to add vitamin D to bread, but, for a number of technical reasons, this failed. It's true that nearly all children eat bread, but there's another food that every child absolutely needs in order to develop strong bones. This, of course, is milk, and it's an even more appropriate vehicle for vitamin D than bread because absorption of the vitamin is more effective in a substance that also delivers fat, and even modern-day low-fat milk contributes some fat to the diet. By 1935, after vitamin D was added to milk the incidence of rickets declined from over 20 percent to barely detectable levels. Milk bolstered with vitamin D ranks among the liquid triumphs of nutritional science.

Rickets has, for all practical purposes, been eliminated in affluent countries through the fortification of milk. However, the disease would reappear if the supplementation were omitted. In the 1950s Scotland learned this lesson when the government decided that butter alone would be an adequate source of vitamin D, and stopped fortifying the milk supply. Within a few years the medical profession began reporting an alarming incidence of rickets, and the milk program was restored.

Rickets still persists in England, where there are many immigrants who come from countries where drinking milk is uncommon and the sun is so high in the sky and so bright that the smallest amount of skin exposure is sufficient. But in England, which is in a northern latitude and has much inclement weather, the level of ultraviolet light is much lower and requires exposure of a larger area of skin than these people, especially the women, are accustomed to.

Whether taken as a supplement or activated by sunlight falling on the skin, vitamin D functions in several ways to develop and maintain strong, well-formed bones. Before looking closely at rickets and at related diseases in adults, it will be helpful to understand normal bone function.

O Dem Bones

Bones consist of calcium and phosphorus set in a protein matrix called collagen. The word is based upon a root meaning "glue" —a boiled bone literally does yield glue—but collagen should be regarded less as an adhesive that holds calcium and phosphorus together than as a structure within which these rigid bone materials are found.

Vitamin D is essential for calcium absorption. When sunlight strikes the skin the vitamin is activated, then converted into a material that transports calcium across the intestinal wall into the bloodstream. Along with calcium, this material also, to some extent, helps the body absorb phosphorus. Vitamin D works with other hormones to help regulate calcium distribution in the body.

This entire process is relevant not only to growing children but to adults as well. Throughout life, cells are constantly being replaced and calcium is being released into the blood and flushed out of the body. Calcium needs to be replaced throughout the life span, and this can happen only with the help of vitamin D. If we are deficient in vitamin D, we cannot absorb enough calcium even if dietary sources are adequate. The result in adults is osteomalacia, or soft bones. This is not to be confused with osteoporosis, a condition caused not mainly by a lack of vitamin D, but by other factors, including a lack of calcium in the diet (see Chapter 7).

Osteomalacia occurs most frequently among women in less-developed countries during pregnancy and lactation. If a woman stays indoors, becomes deficient in vitamin D, and thus can't absorb dietary calcium, her body borrows the mineral from her bones. The alveolar bone, the lower jawbone that supports the teeth, is one of the first tissues to give up its calcium. Teeth loosen and the gum becomes infected, resulting in loss of teeth. The vertebrae in the back also have a spongy matrix somewhat similar to (although not the same as) the alveolar bone. Low back pain can result from lifelong dietary calcium inadequacies and numerous pregnancies.

A level of vitamin D sufficient to sustain a woman prior to pregnancy may be too low once she is carrying a baby. The reason is that the offspring benefits at the expense of the parent. If the mother does not absorb sufficient dietary calcium to provide for the baby's needs, either while it's in the womb or while she's breast feeding, the mother's body will begin reabsorbing calcium from its own bones and supplying it to the child. If this happens the mother needs a good supply of vitamin D (and/or calcium) to replace what has been lost. Otherwise she can suffer permanent bone damage.

Children are especially vulnerable to a vitamin D deficiency because their bones are developing fast—an infant doubles its size in the first year—whereas adult bones only need to maintain their integrity. Since bone growth involves proper mineralization of bone, one result of deficiency—or rickets—in children is bowlegs. Likewise, the ribs may fail to develop adequately, and even the skull can be malformed. At its worst, this disease can result in death; at a more subtle level rickets can be restricted to poor joint formation, which can be detected only through extensive x-ray analysis by a competent orthopedic expert.

Although rickets was first identified in 1650, very little was known about the disease until the late nineteenth century, when scientists extensively studied the bones of children who had died from the disease. Between about 1890 and 1920 researchers began to rediscover what the wives of Weistar had somehow known: rickets could be avoided by exposure to sunlight. They further found that even artificial light could help if it was rich in the ultraviolet rays. It was not until 1922 that scientists proved that the anti-ricketic effect of cod-liver oil was dependent not upon vitamin A, as it was thought, but upon some other factor. They did this by oxidizing the oil, knowing that vitamin A is destroyed by oxidation. Whatever was preventing rickets must be invulnerable to this process, as vitamin D turned out to be.

Excess Vitamin D and Toxicity

Although we have been focusing on vitamin D deficiency, excessive amounts can cause problems as well, as in the case of vitamin A. It is important to stay within the optimum range, which means we should consume neither too little nor too much. The U.S. government recommends 400 International Units of vitamin D per day. If a person consumes over 2000 units—five times the recommended level—for a long period, the body absorbs correspondingly excessive amounts of calcium, which then has to be excreted, placing a strain upon the kidneys. If the strain is severe, the kidneys can fail, resulting in death.

Short of death, toxicity symptoms include diarrhea, headache, and nausea; and if overdose continues to occur, calcium deposits can form in the soft tissues of the body as the vitamin mobilizes too much mineral from the bone. Obviously, this can happen most easily in infants, whose overzealous mothers may go by the rule that if something is good, a little more is better. Vitamin D toxicity is somewhat insidious in the sense that it is very rarely observed and thus physicians may miss it as they seek other causes for the vague symptoms that I've described. Thus, vitamin D toxicity is something to be carefully avoided.

Vitamin D in the Twentieth Century

In the world of the late twentieth century, vitamin D is taken for granted. In some places the main source is the sun, but in much of the North, for at least part of the year, we rely mainly upon the vitamin D added to milk or provided through supplementation. Think about why this is so. A person can live in a Chicago apartment, travel to New York for a meeting, go out for dinner and return home, all without going out into the sunlight at all. Hotels have covered atriums or interior lobbies, airports have underground parking and covered areas where taxis can pull up. Schoolchildren spend most of their day in the classroom, are often taken to and from school in automobiles or buses and have other indoor activities in late afternoon. Even their exercise is often taken inside a large gymnasium. If TV sets could activate vitamin D, most of us would never have to worry about our supply, but during the four to eight hours that many people watch TV they are seldom doing so in the sun.

It is true that we have a cult of the suntan, at least for a quarter or a third of the year, and, for those who can afford the luxury of a plane to the Caribbean or Hawaii, in the winter as well. But recently we have been sternly warned about the risk of skin cancer from excessive exposure to ultraviolet light. Instead of settling for moderate exposure, some people are now going to the other extreme and avoiding the sun as much as possible.

To provide optimum vitamin D it would be nice if we could provide measured and convenient indoor sources of ultraviolet light, especially for people who are institutionalized, who work in offices, or who stay indoors all day. One could even imagine a law that would require that a certain quota of artificial sunlight be available to office workers or schoolchildren under all conditions. However, this would involve yet another set of regulations. It would be more expensive than a vitamin D supplement and it would not necessarily create an automatic link with the ingestion of calcium.

We are back to the question of dietary sources. Like vitamin A, vitamin D is an animal product, but it cannot be made by the body from a vegetable source in the same way that vitamin A can be created by beta-carotene. Vitamin D is found in dairy products, such as milk, cream, and butter, in eggs, and in organ meats such as livers and kidneys. Oily fish is an especially rich source. In northern Europe the need for vitamin D may have been part of the reason for the Catholic practice of eating fish every Friday.

Is Supplementation an Answer?

People who fail to drink an adequate supply of milk and to have regular exposure to the sun need to supplement their diet with vitamin D. Otherwise they risk the same difficulties that faced people of thirteenth-century Weistar—the inability of the body to form and thereafter maintain well-formed, resilient bones.

As more and more of the population pay attention to various dietary dangers, foods rich in vitamin D are decreasing in popularity. Eggs also contain cholesterol, which is related to heart disease. Butter is giving way to margarine, which is sometimes fortified with vitamin D, but not always. Although we still eat a diet heavy in fats, these are increasingly derived from vegetable sources, which are devoid of vitamin D. Most serious of all is the decline in the consumption of milk because, unlike eggs and butter, it also contains a substantial supply of calcium.

Many people need to take calcium supplements. In fact, it is probably important for every woman to use a calcium supplement regularly from about the age of fifteen. If she doesn't get enough vitamin D, either from the sunlight or from dietary sources, she will require adequate vitamin D in order to absorb the calcium. Therefore, if she doesn't eat foods rich in vitamin D or get plenty of sunlight she should be sure to get 400 International Units of vitamin D each day from a supplement. A good multivitamin or multimineral should contain that. As we've seen, excessive amounts of vitamin D are to be avoided.

Is Vitamin D Really a Vitamin?

The strange thing about vitamin D is that, since the human body can make its own supply, it may not qualify as a vitamin at all. Apart from dietary cholesterol, the liver makes all the cholesterol the body needs; some of it is carried by the blood to the skin, where, struck by the ultraviolet rays of the sunlight, it is converted to vitamin D. The vitamin is then further converted by the kidneys and the liver into active forms that help the body to absorb calcium and deposit it where it belongs. In this process, both the cholesterol and the vitamin D are made by the body itself. All that's required from the outside is sunlight. That's why vitamin D is regarded as the sunshine vitamin. Only when we fail to spend adequate time in the sun do we need to ingest vitamin D at all.

4

VITAMINS E AND K

Claims and Facts

Spanish explorer Ponce de León spent years searching the Caribbean for the fabled fountain of youth. He never found it. Nor has anyone else. Yet today some people go Ponce de León one better. They claim to have found the secret not only of eternal youth but of sexual potency too, all in one single nutrient: vitamin E.

Over the last two decades vitamin E has been sold as the stud of vitamins. Rumor has it that this fat-soluble vitamin heightens sexual vigor, strengthens athletic power and endurance, cures heart ailments, and prevents aging. Unfortunately, none of these claims holds up under the scrutiny of science.

Ever since its discovery, E has been a vitamin in search of a disease. As we begin to understand vitamin E's functions better we can see exciting roles supplemental vitamin E might play in human health. But first, like Ponce de León, we must do a little exploring.

Of Rats and Men

From the very beginning nutritional science has changed and changed again its theories on how vitamin E works. In 1922, the vitamin was identified as a key factor in the fertility of rats. When rats were deprived of it, they could not reproduce. So, when vitamin E was finally isolated in 1936, its association with reproduction led to its being named "tocopherol" meaning in Greek to give birth.

During the next decade, other dramatic vitamin E deficiency symptoms were found in animals—heart damage in calves, retarded growth in rabbits, liver degeneration and muscular dystrophy in chicks and rabbits. There was great hope that similar ailments in humans were also caused by vitamin E deficiency so that supplying the vitamin would make the ailments disappear.

No such luck. No deficiency or deficiency diseases were ever found in humans. The government even went so far as to keep volunteers on a low vitamin E diet for six years beginning in 1953. They were watched closely for physical or mental effects. Nothing happened.

People afflicted with muscular dystrophy were tested. It turned out that their tissues contained as much vitamin E as those of people without the disease. Thus, there is no evidence that muscular dystrophy in humans is associated with vitamin E deficiency.

In 1970 one scientist put it, "Vitamin E is one of those embarrassing vitamins that has been identified, isolated and synthesized by physiologists and biochemists and then handed to the medical profession with the suggestion that a use should be found for it." All the claims, emotions, and counterclaims surrounding vitamin E intrigued scientists. They suspected that this vitamin indeed had important uses that they just hadn't understood yet. Now, finally, the answers are coming into focus.

Vitamin E: What Is It?

Vitamin E is actually a complex of eight substances: four tocopherols and four tocotrienols. They are thick light yellow oils, insoluble in water, resistant to heat, but readily destroyed by ultraviolet light (sunlight, for example), freezing, and prolonged exposure to air.

The four substances to keep in mind are the tocopherols, named for the first four letters in the Greek alphabet—alpha, beta, gamma, delta. Although the exact effectiveness of the other tocopherols has not been established, it appears that alpha-tocopherol is responsible for 80 percent of vitamin E activity.

How Vitamin E Works

Unlike most other vitamins, vitamin E does not help break down food or energy. It does not function as a co-enzyme in metabolism like vitamins A, C, and the B complex. Vitamin E does become involved in energy metabolism, but only after it's over. And we are very fortunate that it does.

Oxygen in the body burns food for energy, just as it burns wood for fuel in the fireplace or gasoline for fuel in the engine. In the body, the other vitamins help this happen. We say that the food is "oxidized." But sometimes oxygen doesn't stop there. Even after a metabolic reaction has taken place, some oxygen molecules continue to break things down. They have no "off" switch. Once fuel is "burned," oxygen molecules generate destructive compounds that attack cells and cell membranes. If unchecked, these "free radicals" can destroy nutrients stored in cells and cause cell damage.

Fats and the essential fatty acids that make them up are particularly vulnerable to oxidation. This is true not only in the body but in foods as well. No doubt you've had a bottle of oil or a bag of potato chips turn rancid. That rancidity is the effect of oxidation on the fatty acids in the vegetable oils. These are usually unsaturated oils—liquid at room temperature unless artificially hardened by hydrogenation.

Vitamin E comes to the rescue. It is a powerful antioxidant. That's why it's found naturally in polyunsaturated oils. It acts as a kind of scavenger for the destructive substances that would otherwise react with the oil's unsaturated bonds and cause decomposition. Scientists recently learned that a trace mineral, selenium, works together with vitamin E in such a way that one enhances the antioxidant activity of the other.

Vitamin E acts as an antioxidant in the body, too. It protects the polyunsaturated fats in all the cell membranes of the body. These fatty components of the body may go "rancid"—that is, undergo oxidation—just like other fats and oils. Supplies of vitamin E are distributed throughout the body. Each of our trillions of cells contains some vitamin E in the fatty cell membranes.

While it is one of the most effective natural antioxidants in the world, vitamin E is not inexhaustible. If continuously bombarded by enormous amounts of oxygen, it can be overwhelmed and oxidized itself. That's why you need to put the cap back on the bottle of oil—and why it's a good idea to maintain optimum levels of vitamin E in your body.

If you increase the amount of polyunsaturated fats in your diet, you increase your need for vitamin E. In most cases, this works out because they occur in the same foods. But, if you eat many foods like frozen french fries or doughnuts that are high in these fats but have lost their vitamin E, you need to increase your intake of vitamin E–rich foods.

Vitamin E and Premature Infants

Because of its antioxidant function, vitamin E helps doctors save the lives of premature infants, many of whom are anemic. They simply haven't had the time to build iron-rich red blood cells, which transport oxygen.

At one time doctors tried improving premature infants' oxygen intake by giving them iron. The infants' bodies were less able to cope with oxidation triggered by the oxygen because they had low levels of vitamin E. Vitamin E levels in fetuses are low in the first and second trimesters of pregnancy and don't increase until the third trimester. Without adequate vitamin E, the membranes of the red blood cells were weakened and the cells were destroyed.

Adding vitamin E to the iron supplement helped solve the problem. It enabled pre-term infants to receive the high concentrations of iron they need to survive with less risk of oxidation damage.

It was this discovery in 1965 that helped to illuminate vitamin E's antioxidant function. Premature infants were the first humans discovered to be suffering from a lack of this vitamin. In trying to help them, scientists learned some of the ways in which vitamin E sustains human health.

Some scientists believe that it is because levels of vitamin E in premature infant cell membranes are low that exposure to rich oxygen supply can cause eye damage, even blindness. But, if doctors use supplemental vitamin E, this type of oxidation may be preventable. More research is called for in this area.

Human milk is rich enough in vitamin E to meet normal infant needs. Supplemental vitamin E is required only for formula-fed infants, especially those born prematurely. In any case, no supplemental vitamin should be given to any infant without the guidance of a physician.

Vitamin E, Cystic Fibrosis, and Sickle Cell Disease

Besides premature infants, people who cannot absorb fats provide the only other known examples of human vitamin E deficiency. Patients with cystic fibrosis often have great difficulty absorbing vitamin E, which is fat-soluble, as well as other fats and fat-soluble vitamins. Lack of vitamin E's antioxidant protection may mean shortened red-blood-cell survival. To extrapolate from red cells to other tissues is a big jump. Nevertheless, evidence indicates the same oxidation effects might be going on in other tissues.

Recently, vitamin E has also been shown by Dr. Clayton Natta to be low in patients with sickle cell anemia. Sickle cell disease predisposes red blood cells to oxidative damage. In this study, ten out of thirteen sickle cell anemia patients were found to be deficient in vitamin E.

Theories on Vitamin E and Aging

Major scientific discoveries do not occur in isolation. Usually there are many scientists converging on the same problem. It's just a matter of who finds the answer first. When vitamin E's antioxidant ability came to light some people thought, "Aha, what's growing old but oxidation of tissue? Perhaps here's the pill that will protect us from the ravages of old age." But we must ask ourselves, if something as monumental as a way to stop human aging has been found, why has it not been seized upon by scientists everywhere? That kind of information surely would not be neglected if it were relevant.

Aging, however, is such a complex, lengthy process and the theory about the effects of vitamin E is at such an early stage that no definite statements can yet be made. In tests performed on mice, enormous amounts of vitamin E were unable to slow the decline in function due to aging. Because the process of human aging is so gradual, the theory will remain just that—a theory—for quite some time.

Can Vitamin E Protect Us from Pollution?

Take a deep breath. If you're like most Americans, you live in a bustling metropolitan or suburban area and you've just inhaled a noxious soup that includes nitrogen dioxide and ozone. Once inside your lungs, these chemicals react with fatty acids to generate harmful free radicals. Once this process starts, it becomes a chain reaction.

As environmental pollution worsened in the last few decades, many scientists examined vitamin E's antioxidant functions. They hoped to find some biochemical armor against pollution. Since the 1970s an increasing number of scientists have come to believe that vitamin E's gift to modern health could be its antioxidant protection against air pollution.

Because scientists can't very well set up experiments to expose human subjects to harmful substances, data on vitamin E and pollution in humans are limited. But studies in numerous laboratories on several species of animals show that vitamin E has a very definite effect on the survival of those exposed to either ozone or nitrogen dioxide.

Animals with low vitamin E levels are three to ten times as sensitive to pollution effects as animals given large amounts of vitamin E supplements. This has not been shown to be the same for humans. However, in one of the few human studies on vitamin E and pollution done by Dr. A. L. Tappel, ten subjects were exposed to the pollutant ozone while bicycling in a controlled environment. Large amounts of vitamin E were found to lower the level of oxidation by-products present in the subjects' expired breath.

Many of the basic features of these tests are similar enough to conditions affecting urban people to warrant our applying the results to humans. Vitamin E and other antioxidants to be discussed later may be among the most important defense systems we have against oxidant lung injury from the polluted air we breathe.

The Myth of Vitamin E and Sex

How did vitamin E get its undeserved reputation as the sex vitamin? When lack of vitamin E became associated with sterility in male rats and miscarriage in female rats, some people leaped to the hope that vitamin E supplements would cure human sterility. And, once vitamin E and sex were linked in people's minds, it was only a short step to credit vitamin E with improving virility and sexual stamina.

Recall, though, that the rats' reproductive problems leading to the discovery of vitamin E were the result of total deprivation of vitamin E for an extended time. It is unlikely that any human diet could possibly be deficient enough to lead to such severe problems.

Admittedly, research in this area is complicated. For one thing, it is difficult to conduct the appropriate tests on humans that are needed for scientific proof. For another, so much of human sexuality is psychological that we must take into account the placebo effect. If somebody believes something will work, it may work. The placebo effect is so strong that in most bona fide clinical tests on nutrients and medications, scientists arrange to have some subjects given an identical "dummy" pill so that no one, including the experimenter, knows who has the real thing. Hence no one's confidence in the treatment will skew the results. So far as we can tell, however, vitamin E has no proven value in preventing sterility or miscarriage in humans.

Vitamin E and Athletes' Ability

Who becomes a real quarterback and who becomes an armchair quarterback is primarily a matter of genetic destiny. Of course, nutrition plays a role. Without optimum nutrition, genetic potential may never reach full bloom.

Athletes may need more of certain nutrients than the average person. For example, scientific evidence indicates that some athletes require more B vitamins or iron. Based on these nutrients' functions, that makes sense. No evidence so far, however, supports the idea that great intakes of vitamin E increase physical vigor, strength, and endurance.

Vitamin E may best serve the athlete who lives, trains, or competes in a polluted urban environment. It seems likely that supplemental vitamin E may to some extent neutralize the toxic effects of air pollutants that the athlete must inhale in big gulps.

Vitamin E, Circulation, and Leg Pains

In the mid-1940s the belief emerged that vitamin E could cure most heart ailments. Entire clinics devoted to this idea opened. Even though this belief persists somewhat today, the scientific evidence behind it is questionable.

In a half-dozen studies, patients with chronic chest pains and hypertensive and arteriosclerotic heart disease were given vitamin E and placebos. No positive effects of vitamin E were observed.

Dr. K. Haeger and other scientists have found that supplemental vitamin E relieves leg muscle pains, primarily in the calves. This is usually referred to as "claudication pain," most often caused by a narrowing of the arteries in the legs. The question of whether vitamin E has an effect on circulation is unresolved.

Vitamin E and Fibrocystic Breast Disease

Another vitamin E puzzle is its beneficial effects on fibrocystic breast disease. Also known as benign cystic mastitis, this disease has frightened many women who find painful lumps in their breasts. Some experts believe that substances found in coffee, cola, and chocolate cause the cysts. But more evidence points to a hormonal imbalance. Somehow, vitamin E may alter hormone levels to resolve the problem.

Various studies have shown some clinical improvement in women with this condition. However, this is a very complicated disease and any kind of therapy should be supervised by a physician. Future studies will continue to investigate this issue.

What Foods Contain Vitamin E?

If we examine nutrition folklore and food customs around the world, we find no folk traditions for obtaining vitamin E. There is nothing handed down through generations to ensure ample vitamin E in the diet, as is the case with nearly every other vitamin and most minerals. This tells us something—vitamin E is not difficult to get from food. In fact, vitamin E abounds in the diet. The richest sources include grains, nuts, seeds, and beans as well as the oils made from them.

Wheat germ oil is the best natural source, providing about 28 IU per tablespoon. The recommended dietary allowance (RDA) for adults is 12 to 15 IU. Whole grains and leafy green vegetables are also good sources. A few oils, such as corn oil, are relatively high in gamma-tocopherol, not alpha-tocopherol, and therefore poorer than other oils in contributing active vitamin E to the diet. Consuming a variety of oils and natural foods usually ensures meeting RDA levels.

In a typical American diet, about 65 percent of vitamin E comes from salad oils, shortening, margarine, and other fats and oils. But a refined diet that excludes whole grains and fresh vegetables may not provide the RDA for vitamin E. For example, as much as 80 percent is lost when whole wheat is converted to white bread. Freezing vegetables causes some vitamin E destruction as does deep-fat frying foods for long periods of time.

Even with these cooking, processing, and storing methods, you'll still undoubtedly ingest enough vitamin E to get by. Although this will avoid deficiencies, it may not be sufficient to produce the full benefits vitamin E is capable of providing.

Vitamin E Supplementation

Modern science giveth and taketh away when it comes to vitamin E. We can say good-bye to visions of lifelong youth and sexual enhancement from this vitamin. That was myth. But in its place we have a new hope. Vitamin E may help protect us from the pollution that continues to permeate the air we breathe.

Any healthy person who has no difficulty absorbing fats receives enough vitamin E to get by, but it makes sense for many of us to take advantage of the extra protection this powerful antioxidant may provide.

Vitamin K: The Forgettable Vitamin

Here's a vitamin most of us can afford to forget. The need for vitamin K is small—70 to 140 micrograms per day for adults. Our own intestinal bacteria produce much of what we need, and the rest comes from our diet. An average diet along with this bacterial action appears to provide 300 to 500 micrograms daily, at least three times what we need.

What Does Vitamin K Do?

As often happens in science, two separate teams of scientists, one in Denmark and one in California, independently discovered vitamin K within a few months of each other in 1936. Without this substance, chickens could not form blood clots and developed severe hemorrhage problems. Vitamin K was isolated in pure form from alfalfa in 1939.

Since this fat-soluble vitamin proved to be essential to

proper coagulation of blood, the Danish scientists proposed it be called vitamin K for *koagulation,* the Danish and German spelling of the word.

In typical healthy individuals, vitamin K works in the liver to form at least six different proteins necessary for blood clotting. The best known of these is prothrombin.

Vitamin K in Foods

If you want further proof that vitamin K is not a problem for most of us, here it is. The foods that are rich in vitamin K are liver and green leafy vegetables, such as spinach, kale, turnip greens, dark green lettuce, broccoli, cauliflower, and cabbage. These are not the kinds of foods that most people eat every day. Also very little vitamin K is present in most cereals, fruits, carrots, peas, peanuts, oils, most meats, and highly refined foods. Yet there are no vitamin K deficiencies in a normal healthy population.

Who Needs to Worry About Vitamin K?

People who have difficulty absorbing fats may need vitamin K supplements. This is for a doctor to decide.

In newborn infants, particularly premature infants, intestinal bacteria may not have become established yet. If this is the case, doctors may give infants vitamin K as a precaution.

Antibiotics knock out bacteria, good with bad, so prolonged use of this type of medication can pose a vitamin K problem. In that case, you may wish to take vitamin K in some form, with your doctor's supervision.

Introduction to the Water-Soluble Vitamins

JULIAN SPALLHOLZ, PH.D.

Nutritional practices that have been passed through generations for hundreds of years are the empirical results of people's seeking better health and freedom from disease. The discovery of organic factors required in the diet in rather small amounts, the compounds we collectively call vitamins, is by any historical measure a contemporary event.

The vitamines (sic) and growth-related factors that were isolated from foods in the earlier part of this century were initially separated based upon their solubility in either oils (fat) or water. The water-soluble vitamins of the B group were at the time designated by subscript numerals following terminology introduced early on by British biochemists. By 1920, E. V. McCollum (1879–1967), working at the University of Wisconsin, had identified a fat-soluble A and a water-soluble B vitamine. When ascorbic acid was incorporated into the vitamine scheme of things at the time, it finished third (vitamin C) in a growing vitamine alphabet.

Today we recognize vitamin C and eight members of a vitamin B complex as the essential dietary water-soluble vitamins. Thiamin (vitamin B_1) was first isolated in 1926. Riboflavin (vitamin B_2), variously known as lactoflavin, ovoflavin, and hepatoflavin according to its source, was initially called vitamine G (for growth) and was separate from vitamin B in 1933. Niacin, pyridoxal (vitamin B_6), biotin, and pantothenic acid were individually isolated between

1935 and 1938. During the forties, folic acid (1945) and cyanocobalamine (vitamin B_{12}) were each isolated and chemically identified. Through the years other vitamin-like factors have been isolated. Once thought to be vitamins, compounds such as choline, p-aminobenzoic acid, inositol, lipoic acid, vitamin M (for monkey), vitamin P (for permeability), and co-enzyme Q (for ubiquinone) were found not to be vitamins for humans. More recently, laetrile and pangamic acid have been designated as vitamin B_{17} and vitamin B_{15}, but they are not vitamins at all.

The vitamins of the B complex and vitamin C are water soluble. Unlike the fat-soluble vitamins (Chapters 2, 3, and 4), they are not appreciably stored in the body. They must be continuously supplied from the diet. Excretion, and their subsequent depletion in the absence of dietary sources, can be rather rapid. This accounts for the historical onset of scurvy in sailors at sea, beriberi in the Javanese, and pellagra in the southern United States when the vitamins were absent or minimally present in the diet.

Two of the water-soluble vitamins, riboflavin (vitamin B_2) and vitamin C, are very susceptible to destruction under certain conditions of light, alkalinity, and temperature. Thus proper storage, processing, and cooking of foods are important factors in retaining viable vitamins in many foods. Vitamin-fortified foods together with balanced vitamin-mineral supplements help prevent dietary deficiencies and the associated nutritional diseases once prevalent in large segments of undernourished and improperly fed people.

5

VITAMIN C

From Limeys to Linus

"An army," Napoleon once said, "marches on its stomach." Yet history focuses on the strategy and logistics of battles won or lost, lands conquered, and discoveries made. It seldom tells about the nutritional conditions that played a part in shaping those events.

During the Crusades of the Middle Ages, thousands of men left the fields of Europe to march to the Middle East. Most of them never made it to Jerusalem, and the goal of the Crusades, to conquer the Islamic nations, was never achieved. When supplies of fresh fruits and vegetables became scarce, great numbers of Crusaders perished from scurvy, a disease that, as we now know, was caused by a lack of vitamin C. Even back home in Europe, whenever crops failed and famine occurred, scurvy contributed to the death toll.

During the great age of seafaring when Spain and England competed on the seas, more sailors were lost to scurvy than to battles or typhoons. For example, when the Portuguese explorer Vasco da Gama made his famed voyage around the Cape of Good Hope at the end of the fifteenth century, nearly two-thirds of his crew perished from scurvy. At the same time, the Italian Amerigo Vespucci was on his way to the Americas. Instead of keeping sick crew aboard and letting them die, he put them ashore on an island inhabited by friendly natives, who gave the sailors fresh fruit. Months later, when the now healthy sailors sought passage home on a Portuguese ship, their recovery was thought to be so miraculous that the island was named Curaçao, which means "cure."

Scurvy is one of humanity's oldest diseases. Accounts date back to 1500 B.C. Aristotle described it in detail about 450 B.C., noting such symptoms as lack of energy, bleeding, inflamed gums, and tooth loss. With impeccable Aristotelian logic, the great philosopher reasoned that, if figs brought about tooth decay as he had discovered, then something else in the diet must cause tooth loosening and gum bleeding. He did not realize that this slow, painful illness was the result of something *missing* from the diet.

Rose Hips, Bark Tea, Raw Fish

While the population of Europe lived at the mercy of an unsteady supply of fresh fruits and vegetables, other cultures in various parts of the world had developed ways to supplement their diets with enough vitamin C to avoid scurvy.

In some of the cold northern regions of the ancient world such as China, Mongolia, Siberia, and Scandinavia, people harvested rose hips—the fruits of the wild rose, a flower found widely in cool climates. They would dry these fruits, grind them into a powder, then make the powder into tea or soup and add it to other foods throughout the long winter months. Even in recent times this old custom stood the Swedes in good stead when their supplies of citrus fruits from Italy and Spain were cut off during World War II. *Nypon sopa* or rose-hip soup was their primary source of vitamin C until the war was over and trade with the South resumed.

Other plants also yield a supply of the anti-scurvy vitamin. In the West Indies, for example, people relied on a kind of cherry called acerola, and in the evergreen forests of North America, natives brewed a vitamin C–rich tea from the tips of spruce needles. In 1535, when the French explorer Cartier became trapped in Canada during a heavy winter, he and the men on his expedition were helped to survive by learning to make this brew. Likewise, missionaries who went to live with tribes in lower Canada and the northern plain states were in danger of developing scurvy during the winter months. Some adapted to the native diet and brewed their tea from bark and needles recommended by the native Americans. Others persisted in drinking English teas. The former avoided scurvy.

In the case of missionaries who journeyed to Alaska, the remedy was a little harder to take. The Eskimo habit of eating raw fish struck them as heathen. In contrast they scrupulously cooked their fish and tried to make the natives do likewise. As it happens, however, cooking destroys the vitamin C in raw fish, so the missionaries' reward for their zeal was scurvy. Fortunately some of them learned that scurvy could be reversed if they ate the fish the Eskimo way.

Thus we see how different people developed food habits and customs based on observation and ingenuity. Over centuries, they learned to meet nutritional needs with readily available foods or with materials we might not even consider food. Many of these customs, such as using acerola cherries and rose hips as sources of vitamin C, survive today in those parts of the world. Unfortunately, though, waters off populous areas have become too polluted to make unprepared raw fish a safe source.

Lind to the Rescue

The year was 1747 and Britannia ruled the waves. The empire's vast colonies stretched east to India and west to North America. But for the average British sailor life was still fraught with perils. If he set sail on a voyage due to last six months or more, scurvy was almost certain to send him to a watery grave. Almost certain, we say, because some sailors did not get scurvy. Individual differences in vitamin C requirement allowed some to survive, which must have seemed a miracle.

So great were the odds against survival that the captain of a hundred-foot schooner, the *Salisbury,* hired on a crew of eight hundred just to make sure that enough men would be left to steer the ship home after scurvy had taken its loathsome toll. The *Salisbury* had barely reached the Strait of Gibraltar when some of the men started to show the symptoms of scurvy. When the captain ordered, "All hands on deck!" the afflicted men couldn't move quickly. Physical symptoms were even more obvious. When sick crew members ate the hard, dried rations of bread and salt pork, their gums would bleed. They were vulnerable to all kinds of infection, from common colds to ulcerous sores that never healed. Blood vessels broke under the skin surface and appeared as tiny red fissures.

The ship's doctor, a young naval surgeon, could not bear to stand by while the men in his charge sickened and died. Dr. James Lind set out to conquer scurvy.

One night as Lind left the officers' dining room to visit his patients in the mess hall, he noticed that ordinary sailors did not get any of the Brussels sprouts and potatoes the officers received. Since officers did not get scurvy, Dr. Lind wondered whether the fresh vegetables protected them from the disease. Then the *Salisbury* came across a Dutch ship returning from Spain with oranges and lemons. Much to Dr. Lind's amazement, sick men who ate some of the fruit became well. Could something as simple as food cure this disease?

To find out, Lind bought some of the fruit from the Dutch with his own money and set up an experiment that, although simple, launched modern nutrition research. He selected twelve scurvy-sick sailors and divided them into two groups of six. Lind cooked all their meals himself to make sure each group ate an identical diet except for one item. Within six days the men who had received citrus fruit recovered.

Although for centuries alchemists and witch doctors had boasted of magic potions that they claimed would cure scurvy, Dr. Lind's study provided a simple, indisputable answer. But his pleas to provide enlisted sailors with fresh fruit fell on deaf ears. The Royal Navy did nothing for nearly fifty years. But famed voyager Captain James Cook read Lind's work and prevented scurvy on his ship by putting in a supply of fruit. It wasn't until 1795, ironically one year after Lind's death, that the Royal Navy ordered each sailor to be provided with a ration of lime juice, and thus the British sailors received their popular nickname, "limeys."

What was in the fruit that prevented scurvy? Today we know it was vitamin C. But nearly two hundred more years had to pass before scientists were able to isolate pure crystals of vitamin C from lemon juice.

Unfortunately, scurvy continued to claim victims. Many westering American pioneers died of it before reaching California, where the Spanish-built missions abounded with citrus trees. As recently as World War I troops died of scurvy, sharing the fate of so many of the Crusaders.

Scurvy's Symptoms

In 1912, scientists started to refer to what they called the "scurvy vitamine" or "antiscorbutin" because it was "antiscorbutic" (prevented scurvy). In 1932, when the substance in fruits that prevented scurvy was identified, "antiscorbutic" was shortened to "ascorbic" and the new vitamin was named "ascorbic acid." This was shortened again to vitamin C.

Determining vitamin C's actual functions proved challenging because the symptoms of scurvy are manifested in so many ways. It was apparent that without vitamin C the body literally falls apart. Gums deteriorate and teeth fall out, blood vessels break, cuts don't heal, infections set in.

All this happens because vitamin C is required for the synthesis of certain proteins. Protein is what the body is primarily made of. When you look in the mirror, you're looking at an amazing mosaic of protein. Hair, skin, eyes, muscle—much of you that shows and much of you that doesn't is made up of protein. Blood and lymph, heart and lungs, brain and nerves all are predominantly protein or depend on protein.

Many of the body's trillions of cells are constantly sloughed off and renewed. That takes a lot of energy and that's what some of the food you eat is used for. The process that maintains and renews the body systems by using energy and materials from food is called metabolism.

Coordinating all the reactions involved in metabolism is every bit as complicated as launching a space flight, and the body does it automatically. But if one nutrient is missing or out of balance the whole system is affected.

When a bricklayer builds a wall he uses mortar in between

the bricks to make them stick together. When the body builds tissue it uses a special kind of protein called collagen to make the cells adhere. Collagen is the body's connective tissue. As people age, collagen fibers lose their ability to hold the skin tightly together and the skin sags and creases. When vitamin C is inadequate, the body can't make collagen at all. Tissues that receive the most wear and tear, such as the gums, undergo rapid renewal and are quickest to show signs of deficiency. Hence the bleeding and infected gums of the scurvy sufferer.

Collagen is also essential to strong teeth and bones, parts of the body once thought to consist solely of calcium. Clinical evidence supports vitamin C's role in assuring the integrity of bones and teeth. For example, studies on restoring bone density in elderly women found better results when the women took a multivitamin supplement with calcium than when they took calcium supplements. Very recent studies showed that monkeys on a vitamin C–deficient diet developed more cavities than those on a normal diet. Children who lack adequate vitamin C show less than optimal tooth and bone development—another example that calls to mind the scurvy-sick sailors of yore who lost their teeth and experienced pain in their joints.

When you cut or burn yourself protein tissue is destroyed. A minor cut will usually heal and within a week or two the skin looks as if it had never been cut at all. That's because your body's supply of vitamin C worked overtime to weave new protein fibers into place. In fact, people who have been severely burned or injured may require extra vitamin C to help their bodies heal.

Vitamin C in the Blood

Blood contains many kinds of proteins. Vitamin C helps these proteins perform their tasks, too, and if the diet falls short of vitamin C, these functions will suffer.

Antibodies are important blood proteins because they protect us from infection and disease. The immune system, including antibodies, is the body's main form of defense against the onslaught of viruses such as the one that causes the common cold and against any type of invading bacteria. So many billions of harmful microorganisms surround us that our antibodies are constantly being used and must be renewed very quickly. When vitamin C is insufficient, the immune system's ability to fight germs diminishes.

Capillaries are the tiny blood vessels that transfer blood from the arterial system to the venous system. Vitamin C helps keep the capillaries strong. Without vitamin C they become fragile and hemorrhage at the slightest impact, showing up as purplish bruises or networks of tiny red lines just beneath the skin's surface.

If you've ever seen a serious alcoholic, you may have seen a face crisscrossed with these tiny red lines. Excess alcohol intake may not only increase blood pressure but also interfere with vitamin C absorption. If capillaries are weakened, the combination may result in a change in facial color.

Vitamin C also takes part in the forming of hemoglobin, the most important constituent of the red blood cell, and helps the body to absorb iron, a key component of hemoglobin. It is the iron in hemoglobin that enables the blood system to carry oxygen to all the tissues of the body. In fact, it's the iron in hemoglobin that gives it its red color. When there's not enough iron, the blood can't carry as much oxygen. The result is weakness and fatigue.

A scurvy victim is deficient not only in hemoglobin, which carries oxygen, but also in adrenalin, a hormone that increases the flow of blood. Let's say you're at the movies and someone yells, "Fire!" You may find that you can run faster than you've ever run before. This is because of adrenalin. In a dangerous or tense situation, adrenalin is what gets your heart pumping faster, increasing the blood flow to the brain so you can think fast. It also gives you that extra surge of energy to either confront the situation or run lickety-split in the other direction. We call this the "fight or flight" response. Among its many other benefits vitamin C helps to produce adrenalin. In fact, there is more of this vitamin stored in the adrenal glands than anywhere else in the body. It is vitamin C's role in adrenalin metabolism that may explain why British sailors with scurvy couldn't budge when the captain yelled, "All hands on deck!"

These are the functions of vitamin C we know about conclusively, the ones scientists have noted since the days of Dr. James Lind. But in recent years sophisticated technology has allowed scientists to study vitamin C in new ways and to develop new theories about its functions. While these theories are still controversial I believe they are worth discussing.

Theories on Vitamin C and Cancer

Vitamin C is one of a handful of nutrients in the body now known to be antioxidants. Some oxidation is vital, for example to help break down food for energy, but if unchecked, oxidation can damage cell membranes and cause cell mutations. Since our intake of oxygen is constant so is our need for antioxidants, which step in and save the day when oxygen by-products in the body get out of hand. But in the process, antioxidants such as vitamin C are sometimes destroyed themselves.

To see vitamin C's antioxidant properties in action, try this simple experiment. Slice an apple in half. Sprinkle lemon juice liberally over one of the halves. Expose both halves to the air and watch. In a short time, the half not protected by vitamin C will turn brown.

As we have been warned, bacon, pepperoni, and frank-furters contain nitrates and nitrites that the body may convert into cancer-causing nitrosamines. But did you know that nearly all vegetables and fruits also contain nitrites and have the potential to form nitrosamines? Unlike processed meat, however, broccoli, spinach, cantaloupes, and the like contain vitamin C. Emerging scientific theory holds that vitamin C may neutralize the nitrosamines' carcinogenic potential. If one's intake of vitamin C–rich foods is less than adequate, consumption of meats containing nitrates and nitrites makes cancer of the stomach and the esophagus more likely. At any rate, this is the hypothesis put forth by scientists who suspect a connection between vitamin C and cancer, namely that vitamin C, like a football player blocking his opponent from making a forward pass, may block nitrates and nitrites from forming nitrosamines and may also block other cancer-causing agents.

Theories on Vitamin C and Smoking

It's been demonstrated that smoking cigarettes lowers vitamin C levels in the blood. Tests repeatedly find that smokers have lower plasma levels of vitamin C than nonsmokers. Theory has it that the vitamin C may have been spent defending the body. Although the vitamin C depletion observed in smokers is small and considered inconsequential by some scientists, I believe it is indicative of vitamin C's important antioxidant function. By the way, if you smoke—and I hope you don't—please don't be foolish enough to think that taking vitamin C supplements can overcome all the damage you are doing to your cardiovascular system.

Vitamin C and Colds

If your vitamin C intake is inadequate, your body's immune system is not likely to work at its best.

In recent years some scientists, led by Nobel Prize winner Linus Pauling, put forth the controversial theory that very large amounts of vitamin C can prevent colds. Dr. Pauling's reasoning is based on the fact that most living creatures can synthesize their own vitamin C. When they do, it is in amounts far greater in proportion to body weight than the 60 milligrams recommended by the U.S. Dietary Allowance, sometimes six to ten times as much. Monkeys, who like humans can't make their own vitamin C, have a diet, whether in the wild or in captivity, that is much higher in vitamin C than ours. Thus, Dr. Pauling maintains, humans have a better shot at staving off the common cold and other ills when our vitamin C intake is on a level with that of most other creatures. New evidence that gives some support to this was published recently by Dr. S. Boyd Eaton in a medical journal. Working together with an anthropologist, Dr. Eaton concluded that our prehistoric ancestors consumed an average of 400 milligrams of vitamin C per day. The researchers based their estimate on the vitamin C content of plants known to have formed a large part of the paleolithic diet.

Of course the connection to contemporary people is tenuous and Dr. Pauling's theories are generally opposed by most conservative scientists. Research on the common cold is difficult to conduct because of the myriad of cold viruses. But, although the body of research does not support the hypothesis that vitamin C can prevent colds, there is some preliminary evidence that vitamin C may help diminish a cold's severity. In any case, less than adequate intakes of most nutrients can make you more susceptible to disease.

What Happens When You Get a Chill

Imagine this. You're skiing hard and sweating profusely. After you make it down the mountain, you have to wait for your partner or for the next lift. A chill wind blows through your sweat-soaked garments. You may not realize it, but your antibody protection is taking a nosedive. And, if your tissue supplies of vitamin C aren't what they should be, you are in a state of nutritional stress and may not be able to withstand cold weather.

Some recent studies of young skiers suggest that, when exposed to a sudden drop in temperature, the body's antibody level takes a dive. The antibodies most likely to be affected are those most capable of fighting the viruses that cause colds and flus. The body's ability to rebound quickly with new antibodies depends on its vitamin C level. People who have depleted their vitamin C supplies—whether because of poor diet choices, smoking, recovery from injury, or stressful situations—may be more vulnerable to getting sick after being exposed to a chill than people with ample vitamin C in their systems.

More research needs to be done in this area to clarify exactly who is susceptible to this phenomenon and when. However, the early findings provide another argument in the case against crash diets that force the body into such a depleted state that it can't respond quickly when challenged by germs. Obviously, additional studies are required to quantify and interpret these observations.

Vitamin C Requirements

Cats and dogs make their own vitamin C. Rats make their own vitamin C. Most forms of life have some use for vitamin C, and nearly all of them can make it from a simple sugar called glucose. Only a few species lack the enzyme that would enable them to make this important vitamin: these are humans, apes, monkeys, guinea pigs, a bird called the red-vented bulbul, and the Indian fruit bat. There's an irony here because humans need more vitamin C than any other vitamin.

Some biochemists consider lack of this enzyme an "inborn error of metabolism" and speculate that through mutations some humans are able to synthesize sufficient vitamin C in their bodies. Again, recall those sailors on da Gama's long voyage around the Cape of Good Hope. Some survived scurvy, and a few did not get it at all, even though two-thirds of the crew died from it.

No doubt you too probably know some people who catch cold very easily and others who never seem to get sick at all. Or someone who complains of gums bleeding after flossing and brushing the teeth. The fact of the matter is that we still don't know all there is to know about individual requirements for vitamin C. It may very well turn out that the amount of vitamin C needed varies from person to person like shoe sizes. Some people may need more than others for their immune system and tissue synthesis functions.

Despite differences in individual requirement, governments need to set standards to ensure the health of the general population. These standards have to satisfy the average person's needs.

In the case of vitamin C, scientists had to determine the minimum amount required to avoid scurvy. Research volunteers consumed vitamin C–deficient diets to bring about scurvy. Once scurvy symptoms appeared, the scientists worked backward to calculate the lowest level of vitamin C that would prevent appearance of the symptoms.

The absolute minimum requirement of vitamin C per day to prevent scurvy appears to be only about 10 milligrams. But, to allow for growth and maintenance of tissue and to compensate for losses in food, the Food and Nutrition Board of the National Academy of Sciences set the recommended daily allowance at 60 milligrams for adult males and females. The board recognizes that the allowances may not meet the needs of people when they are sick, injured, or consuming a very poor diet.

Because setting the nutrient standards for the nation is such an immense responsibility, the government can't take chances with any new, not-fully-proven theories. The RDAs must be on the conservative side for safety reasons and take into account only nutrition information that has been proven beyond a shadow of a doubt. But that doesn't mean the RDAs are unchangeable. Quite the opposite is true. The National Academy of Sciences' Food and Nutrition Board wisely revises the RDAs about every five years. The growing evidence on vitamin C indicates that we may see some changes in the vitamin C recommendations in the future.

Do We Get Enough?

Clinical symptoms of scurvy are almost unknown in the United States, which suggests that nearly everyone is somehow absorbing at least ten milligrams of vitamin C per day. But, despite the absence of clinical symptoms of this particular disease, a wealth of evidence from biochemical measurements and food-intake surveys indicates that many people in the United States don't get enough vitamin C to meet the standard requirement of 60 milligrams.

Data from the Nationwide Food Consumption Survey, a gargantuan food-intake study by the government, found that 41 percent of the population did not meet the RDA for vitamin C. Of that number, 26 percent consumed less than 70 percent of what they needed. Other recent surveys show that getting adequate vitamin C is a problem for a significant number of teenage boys, young and middle-aged women, and the elderly.

Part of this shortfall can be attributed to choices. Luckily for us, many processed foods are fortified with some vitamin C and, unlike our more distant ancestors, we have citrus fruits available all year long. However, today we eat less than half as many melons, fresh potatoes, fresh cabbage, and fresh apples as did our grandparents. And even so, the vitamin C that we absorb from our food is less than it originally contained—part is destroyed during storage, processing, and cooking.

Now You "C" It, Now You Don't

Like other water-soluble vitamins, vitamin C in foods is extremely susceptible to destruction. Drying and canning as well as cooking and storing zap a food's vitamin C content.

Commercially canned foods may contain more C than home-canned products if the fruits and vegetables reached the cannery fresh from nearby fields and were heated quickly in vacuum-sealed cans. But, if you discard the juice in which the food was canned, the swiftest canning method in the world won't help because whatever vitamin C remains will have dissolved in the liquid.

Prolonged exposure to air makes dried fruits and vegetables a poor source of vitamin C.

Even fresh food can be risky. Spinach reportedly yields approximately 250 milligrams of vitamin C per three ounces. But this measurement is based on samples fresh from the fields. What happens after it's been trucked hundreds or thousands of miles to your supermarket?

In one study, scientists found that fresh spinach had lost some of its vitamin C content by the time it reached the consumer. Unfortunately, there's no way to judge vitamin C content when choosing a bunch of spinach in the produce department. However, when spinach is picked and quickly frozen, sometimes more of the vitamin is retained; a case where modern food processing has improved rather than undermined the quality of our diets.

Vitamin loss doesn't stop when you get the produce home. Peeling produce, chopping it to bits, boiling it in an uncovered pot in water that you later pour down the drain—all detract from the vitamin C available to you and your family. Further loss occurs if the food is prepared in copper, mashed, left in a hot place, or exposed to the air.

Clearly, a high fraction of vitamin C is destroyed in restaurants and institutions where food is usually left on steam tables for hours. A study of five institutions, ranging from school cafeterias to hospitals, found that whipped potatoes had lost 36.2 percent of their vitamin C content after being kept hot for only one hour. Actual serving conditions may require even longer times on the steam table. Findings like these have raised serious concerns about whether hospital patients are getting the vitamin C they urgently need for antibody and collagen synthesis.

To get more vitamin C from produce, buy fruits and vegetables in small quantities and eat them unpeeled and fresh or steamed in a tightly covered pot. Make sure your supermarket keeps the produce on crushed ice or in refrigerated cases. Refrigerate all fresh produce immediately. Frozen produce retains vitamin C well if not allowed to thaw too long before cooking.

Vitamin C Insurance

Say that you don't have time to go to the store every day for fresh produce or that your work requires you to eat a lot of restaurant meals or that your children lunch at the school cafeteria or in the nearest fast-food restaurant. Maybe you ought to consider supplementing your diet with vitamin C as the native Americans, Scandinavians and "limeys" have done.

Today we no longer have to grind spruce needles or rose hips into teas in order to get our vitamin C, nor do we have to eat raw fish: scientifically engineered vitamin C supplements are available.

If you supplement your diet just to the recommended dietary allowance level (say 60 or even as high as 100 milligrams), you can be assured of getting the minimum you need no matter what you eat or how it's cooked. If your diet contains 35 to 65 milligrams, you will have taken no more than 100 milligrams in excess of the RDA. Since vitamin C is water soluble, this amount is easily excreted in the urine if that amount exceeds your particular needs. In many cases extra vitamin C within reason can do little harm and perhaps a lot of good. Supplements can thus provide a form of low-cost nutrition insurance, making sure that all types of individual needs are met.

6

THE B VITAMINS

Of Mead and Meat

It is nightfall at a feudal manor somewhere in the depths of the Middle Ages. Seated around a table in the great hall the lord of the manor and his knights quaff their cups of mead. They have just offered a toast to the lord's health. They have also just supplemented their diets with B vitamins.

Mead, the beverage of choice in the Middle Ages, was made by fermenting honey. When taken straight from the hive, honey contained mostly sugar, not much else. But, thanks to the growth of yeast, fermented honey provided medieval folk not only with a good time but with a rich source of B vitamins. Of course, they didn't know about B vitamins, but they knew mead made them feel hale and hearty—even after the buzz was gone. It is probably because of mead that honey still enjoys a reputation as a health-giving food.

Our scene now shifts to a dense forest in ancient Brazil. Large animals are hard to come by and meat is scarce. The local tribes have learned to brew a dark, fermented beverage they find satisfying. It is beer. Not beer as we know it today, but a thicker, low-alcohol version. Men and women drink as much as three gallons a day and children consume the dried yeast left over from the fermentation process. The beer alone provides 25 to 35 percent of each person's B vitamin requirements.

We are now in the heart of the African jungle of long ago. A swift hunter has just speared a lion. It is a muscular animal and its meat will be tough and stringy—except for the inner organs. While these are still warm, the successful hunter devours them. In his view, this organ meat will make him strong, for it will incorporate the spirit of the animal. In the view of modern science, he was ingesting such valuable nutrients as the B vitamins. The vitamins stored in the organ meat enable the hunter's body to tap into energy he didn't know he had. Rituals evolved around the concepts of red meat and strength—rituals that have helped to shape the way we still prize that thick, juicy steak.

Enter the Redneck

Now we move forward several thousand years. It is the summer of 1915. We are in the cotton fields of the American South. More than fifty years have passed since the end of the Civil War, but the South is still devastated. People are desperately poor. Some of them have little to eat except for the corn they grind into meal. Sometimes they add greens, rice, or sweet potatoes.

Some workers are sitting under a cottonwood tree feeling weak and listless. Their foreman is cussing them as lazy good-for-nothings, as "shade tree sitters." They hoist themselves up and go back to picking cotton. But their skin burns badly in the hot sun—a condition that led to the name "redneck."Actually the reddened skin was a sign that these workers and their families and thousands of others were very, very sick. In 1915 at least 200,000 southerners were suffering from this affliction. About 10,000 died from it that year. What caused it? A vitamin B deficiency. But they didn't know that. No one did.

Pellagra: The Three D's

The name of the disease, pellagra, came from Italy, where *pelle agra* meant "rough skin"; the most striking characteristic of the disease was skin that first turned red on exposure to sunlight, then became dark and cracked. Other body tissues hit hard by pellagra include the digestive tract and the brain. A redneck might develop a sore mouth and tongue, inflamed membranes in the digestive tract with bloody diarrhea, and mental disorientation and hallucinations. Doctors nicknamed pellagra "the three D's": dermatitis, diarrhea, and dementia.

No one was more concerned about the epidemic than Dr. Joseph Goldberger, of the U.S. Public Health Service. As Dr. Goldberger journeyed south to find pellagra's cause and cure, hospitals, orphanages, and mental institutions had more victims of the disease than they could handle.

Doctors then thought pellagra was an infectious disease, spread by germs in the midst of poor sanitation. But Dr. Goldberger had a hunch it was something else. When he visited an orphanage, he noticed that the infants and older children were healthy and only children in the middle group had pellagra. The infants got milk regularly and the older children, who had to work, were given some meat. But children in the middle had neither milk nor meat. From this observation Dr. Goldberger realized that pellagra was caused by an incomplete diet, not by germs.

To prove his theory, on May 7, 1915, in the U.S. Pellagra Hospital in Spartanburg, South Carolina, Dr. Goldberger, his wife, Mary, and four assistants performed a very brave experiment. They mixed scalings of skin sores and intestinal wastes from pellagra victims with a little flour and swallowed it. Then they injected each other with the blood of a pellagrous woman. None of them got pellagra, which was very strong evidence that the disease was not infectious.

Thirty years were to pass before the workings of the B vitamins were understood. But in the meantime people were taught to improve their diets. By 1945 acute pellagra cases had disappeared.

Biological Teamwork

The name of the game is human metabolism. The winning team is the B team. These vitamins control all human energy, whether that energy is used to build a bridge, pick cotton, or do a crossword puzzle. When just one B vitamin is missing from the diet, the body's pattern of metabolism is disturbed. Even if all the other raw materials are present, they cannot be fully used unless the B complex is present in its entirety. Cells may be unable to repair themselves with new protein, or cells may starve in the midst of adequate "fuel" because the fuel can't be burned.

The end result is tissue damage. As in the case of the pellagra victims, the damage shows up first in the parts of the body where the B vitamins are the most active. Both skin and intestinal cells are regularly renewed; this may be why diarrhea and dermatitis are two of the signs of a niacin deficiency.

In the body, vitamins cooperate with each other to do particular tasks, and the B vitamins are the epitome of teamwork at the cellular level. Thus deficiency symptoms overlap. Fatigue, for example, occurs when any one of the B vitamins is missing.

In nutrition we always say teamwork is essential. Scientists only started to understand this biological B team in the 1940s. We still don't know all the reactions that occur or, even among the reactions we do recognize, how all the transformations take place. We do know, however, that all the members of the B team are essential for human growth, development, and metabolism.

The Body's Spark Plugs

In one sense the body converts energy the way an automobile does. In an engine, fuel in the form of gasoline combines with oxygen to make the car run. In the body, fuel in the form of food also combines with oxygen so the body can function. This is what metabolism is all about. In the car engine, the mixture of fuel and air is ignited by the spark plugs at a very high temperature. In the body, a roughly analogous role is played by the B vitamins, which help oxygen to combine with derivatives of the food we've eaten. In this limited sense the B vitamins together with various enzymes act as the body's spark plugs. First they help to break down food into its component parts, then to burn most of these components for energy.

Your need for energy is constant. Thinking, lifting an arm, producing urine or sweat—it takes energy not only to accomplish anything, but also just to keep the body alive. Unlike the spark plugs, the B vitamins and enzymes do their jobs without explosions and high temperatures. After all, you couldn't very well walk around with a series of nonstop explosions taking place inside of you. Nor could the body's delicate organs tolerate excessive heat.

The B vitamins help regulate the release of food energy to the body at a slow, steady rate and at a relatively low temperature—98.6° Fahrenheit. Instead of explosions, there is a long sequence of biochemical reactions, which enable the body to function as a "cool engine."

The body synthesizes all the enzymes it needs to run these reactions, drawing upon its biochemical pantry. But, in order to operate, these enzymes require the help of B vitamins, which function as "co-enzymes." The body cannot make its own B vitamins; they must be supplied by the diet in the right amounts.

Let's return to the car analogy for a moment. Your car's fuel tank may be full of premium gasoline. But if just one spark plug is missing the car simply won't run right. Here again, the workings of the body are similar. If just one of the B vitamins is missing or out of balance, the whole chain of energy-burning reactions is disrupted. You may have had plenty to eat, but if your B vitamin intake was imbalanced or inadequate as in the case of the southern workers circa 1915, you won't have a normal amount of energy.

Meet the B Team Members

At first scientists thought there was only one B vitamin. But, after much detailed research, they found by the late 1920s that vitamin B was not one but several related vitamins. In 1927 a biochemist in Alabama suggested the term "vitamin B complex." At that time this family of vitamins was thought to have only three members. Today when we say B complex we mean the eight water-soluble vitamins that human beings require along with vitamin C. They are thiamin, riboflavin, niacin, B_6, B_{12}, folacin, pantothenic acid, and biotin.

Let us sum up the characteristics they share before we look at them separately:

- They function as co-enzymes for the release of energy from food and for nearly every cellular reaction in the body. Think about that. We have trillions of cells and each cell undergoes a myriad of different biochemical reactions. In addition to being essential for normal growth and development, all the B vitamins are necessary for the maintenance of maximum physical fitness and healthy skin, hair, and nerves.
- Absence of any B vitamin for a sufficient length of time causes death.
- B vitamins are easily destroyed by canning, heating, milling, boiling, and other methods of food processing and storing. Some of these vitamins are also sensitive to light.

Rice Hulls and B_1

Thiamin was the first B vitamin to be identified. Sometimes called B_1, it's also known as the "morale vitamin." Thiamin was discovered when a food-refining process led to a fatal illness.

The Dutch who conquered Java in the early 1900s thought they were doing the native people a favor by building mills so they could have white, polished rice like the Europeans. However, the rice husk removed by the mills had been the people's only source of thiamin. Deprived of the husks, they developed a fatal illness called beriberi. The name literally means "I cannot." This signifies the weakness, lassitude, and muscle atrophy that characterize the disease. Even in the early stages the victims lack the energy to work.

Like the American doctors who later faced the pellagra epidemic of 1915, the Dutch doctors thought beriberi was an infectious disease. Vitamins were unknown in 1900. When a Dutch scientist fed an experimental flock of chickens the polished rice, they too developed beriberi. The scientist thought they had become infected. When his thrifty housekeeper supplemented the chickens' diet with rice husks, they became well. In 1913, the Polish chemist Casimir Funk, working in London, successfully repeated the beriberi experiment with pigeons. The vital factor was named "thiamine" (still often so spelled) and caught the imagination of the world as the nutritional missing link—the vital amine! Vital amine became vitamine, and today the word vitamin has come to stand for all of the organic minute nutrition factors essential to life.

Later studies on people who volunteered to go on low-thiamin diets showed that after only ten days the subjects became depressed and irritable, couldn't concentrate, and lacked interest in their work. More critical symptoms followed within a few weeks. Normal health and morale returned when the subjects received thiamin.

Thiamin helps break carbohydrates down into simple sugar molecules called glucose, which is the brain's only source of energy. Glucose also converts to glycogen, our muscles' source of energy. That's why a thiamin deficiency affects both brain and muscle functions.

Today we eat many refined carbohydrate foods that are as depleted of thiamin as the polished rice of Java. Also, products high in sugar, fat, or alcohol demand thiamin from the body's limited supply in order to be metabolized. Yet they contribute no thiamin in return. They get a free ride, so to speak, at your body's expense.

Milk and B_2

B_2 (riboflavin) was the next B vitamin to be isolated. This was extremely difficult. Riboflavin is so sensitive to light that scientists had to work virtually in the dark. Today we still contend with this problem. The clear plastic containers in which many of us buy milk allow light to diminish its riboflavin content. One of the chief sources of riboflavin in our diets, milk can lose 10 to 17 percent of this vital substance under the fluorescent light used in most supermarkets.

Breaking down food energy is riboflavin's chief energy role. The body burns primarily carbohydrates and fat for energy. During a marathon, endurance athletes usually burn more and more fat as the exercise duration increases. Recent studies suggest that people who exercise heavily need extra riboflavin.

Riboflavin can be found in every cell in the body. It is important not only for energy release but for protein synthesis and many other reactions promoting the body's growth and re-pair. Unfortunately, the best dietary sources of riboflavin—milk, liver, and yeast—are not on most people's lists of favorite foods. Enriched cereals, lean meats, poultry, and eggs are good sources. However, studies indicate that today many healthy, well-fed Americans rely on enriched grain products and supplements to help meet their riboflavin needs.

Lime Water and Niacin

Niacin is the B team member that could have prevented many thousands of Southerners from dying or winding up in mental institutions or, at the very least, from suffering skin disease and diarrhea. Niacin is essential to biochemical reactions in the me-tabolism of carbohydrates, fat, and protein for energy. If it is lacking, the cells' energy pathways are completely blocked.

Dependency on cornmeal triggered the pellagra outbreak in the South. Yet in many parts of Latin America corn flour is a staple and there is no pellagra. That is because it is common to soak the corn in lime water, a practice that makes the niacin in corn available to the body.

The body can also make niacin from the essential amino acid tryptophan, which is abundant in eggs, meat, and dairy products. Because these foods were found to cure pellagra, scientists thought perhaps it was caused by protein deficiency. Then someone cured pellagra with yeasts, and niacin was discovered.

Although pellagra is rare today, poor dietary choices can cause marginal deficiencies. Symptoms include nervous irritabil-ity, insomnia, digestive disorders, headaches, and a swollen, red, sore tongue. In children there may be weakness and poor growth.

Building Blocks and B$_6$

Pyridoxine, as B$_6$ is also called, plays the starring role in protein metabolism. It helps break protein down into its component amino acids. Then it works to build new proteins for the body from these amino-acid building blocks. It helps make the so-called nonessential amino acids, the ones that we don't need to ingest because the body is able to synthesize them. It also helps build hormones and red blood cells, and it acts as a catalyst to convert the amino acid tryptophan into niacin. As many as fifty amino-acid reactions require B_6.

B_6 also helps supply glucose to the brain and to the muscles. In case of deficiency, mental depression and muscle weakness can occur. Another of this vitamin's jobs is to metabolize polyunsaturated fatty acids into components needed for cell membrane structure.

Processing food can drastically reduce its B_6 content. The classic B_6 deficiency story took place in 1951. A batch of commercial infant formula lost its B_6 because it was sterilized at an unusually high temperature. Over 300 babies across the United States began to have convulsions. Luckily , an official in the Food and Drug Administration realized what had happened, and the babies recovered with the help of adequate B_6.

We are not as restricted as an infant in our sources of food, nor are we dependent on others to select them. Yet many of us, unwittingly perhaps, tolerate diets dangerously low in B_6. About 75 percent of the B_6 in wheat is lost during the milling of white flour and is not replaced by enrichment. But how many people eat bread and cakes made with whole-wheat flour? Other processed or refined foods that we eat often contain less than half of the B_6 that was present in the food's natural state.

Certain kinds of medication, birth-control pills, excess consumption of alcohol, pregnancy and lactation, and old age all may increase vitamin B_6 needs. Government surveys indicate that about half the population consumes less than 70 percent of the requirement for B_6.

B_{12} and Your Red Blood Cells

Vitamin B_{12} poses a special problem for strict vegetarians. As commendable as a vegetarian diet may be in some respects, there's simply no way to get B_{12} without consuming animal products. B_{12} is the only vitamin not produced by plants in any form. Even yeast, an excellent source of other B vitamins, contains no B_{12}. All animals have microorganisms in their intestines that synthesize all the B_{12} they need—all animals except human beings. It's a persuasive reason for including some milk or eggs or a supplement in any vegetarian regimen.

B_{12} is so crucial to the production of red blood cells that lack of it leads to what used to be called "tired blood." People who have a condition called "pernicious anemia," which results from the lack of an intestinal B_{12}-binding protein called "intrinsic factor," require a lifelong series of B_{12} injections.

All body cells depend on B_{12}, particularly cells in bone marrow that produce red blood cells and those of the nervous system and the digestive tract. The vitamin is important for its role in the synthesis of DNA and RNA. DNA is the genetic blueprint that is stored in the nucleus of every cell and that enables a cell to duplicate itself.

B_{12} deficiency symptoms result primarily in poorly formed red blood cells, indigestion and diarrhea, and damage to the central nervous system. With lack of B_{12} nerve tissue deteriorates, ultimately including the spinal cord.

Spinach and Folic Acid

Unless you're a wheat germ, liver, and brewer's yeast fan or serve spinach and romaine fresh from the garden, you may be one of the many Americans with borderline folic-acid intake.

One of the last B vitamins to be discovered, folic acid or folacin gets its name from *folium,* which is Latin for foliage or leaf. Folic acid was first isolated in pure form from spinach leaves.

Although folic acid abounds in green vegetables and whole-wheat products, many fail to get the daily requirement, even though it is only about one-half of one milligram. Why? Desserts, white flour, fat, and meat (excluding liver) figure heavily in the diet of many Americans, yet none of them contains much folic acid.

Like vitamin B_{12}, folic acid is essential for the formation of the nucleic acids DNA and RNA. Cells cannot divide properly without it.

Folic acid helps break down into amino acids the proteins that we eat. It also helps the body turn some of those amino acids into new proteins, such as those used to build muscle tissue. Here it works together with vitamin C, B$_6$, and B$_{12}$—an example of biological teamwork.

You can see how times of rapid cell division, like pregnancy, would increase the need for folic acid. Turning from the demand side to the supply side, folic-acid intake can suffer when total food intake is diminished as in a reducing diet or in alcoholism. Remember, too, that cooking can also destroy some of the folic acid in vegetables as can inappropriate storage. Always store vegetables in a cool place. Try to cultivate a taste for crisp steamed vegetables, so you can cook them for shorter time periods with a minimal amount of water. Don't boil vegetables excessively and, when possible, use the cooking water in a soup stock or sauce. It's a rich nutrient source.

Pantothenic Acid: The Everywhere Vitamin

Panto comes from the Greek word "all" and pantothenic acid can be found in every cell in every living thing, plant or animal. All whole natural foods contain it, although foods rich in other B vitamins, such as liver and legumes, are especially good sources.

Pantothenic acid works as a co-enzyme with one of the master enzymes of the body. Together they collaborate in the workshop of metabolism, where food is broken down for energy and the elements are then built up again into complicated compounds that the body needs. Pantothenic acid also plays a role in fatty-acid synthesis, red-blood-cell formation, blood-sugar regulation, and the building of antibodies, nerve and brain tissue, and muscle tissue.

Again we have nutritional teamwork. Pantothenic acid in many of its reactions works together with riboflavin, niacin, thiamin, B$_6$, and several minerals.

Processing and freezing destroy this vitamin and lower the content in many people's diets. Foods such as cornflakes, precooked rice, sugar, and shortening contain little. Experimentally created deficiencies in humans produce symptoms such as fatigue, headache, sleep disturbances, stomach aches, and muscle cramps, but deficiencies in a healthy population are practically unknown. Also, a deficiency would take months to develop. So, if you have a headache, don't jump to the very unlikely conclusion that you have a pantothenic-acid deficiency.

White Streaks and Biotin

Until recently, doctors had little concern for biotin because it was thought that the body could make it in sufficient quantities. But upon the advent of intravenous feeding in hospitals, patients developed severe rashes, depression, lethargy, and a loss of hair because the first formula diets did not include biotin. Now we know that although biotin is made in the intestines, we must also get some from our food.

Biotin is also required for releasing energy from carbohydrates and for the synthesis of glycogen for muscle energy, and of fatty acids, protein, and nucleic acids like DNA.

Hair is made up of protein. It's been found that hair growth slows or stops in people who are biotin deficient. In juvenile biotin deficiency, hair growth has been retarded in fact, baldness resulted, and hair was restored by supplementary biotin. In rare cases of severe adult biotin deficiency, hair has turned white; color returned when dietary biotin was provided. But it would take months of extreme deprivation for symptoms such as these to appear. Hair turning gray is a normal part of the aging process for most people and not the result of a biotin deficiency.

Again, biotin is most abundant in foods that are treasure troves of other B vitamins. Liver, yeast, egg yolks, whole grains, nuts, beans, meats, and dairy products are all good sources. An ironic note here: Many people think of a raw egg as being healthful, but actually raw egg white contains a protein that can bind biotin. Cooking egg white prevents this binding action, so go easy on the raw eggs.

B Robbers: Empty Calories

Pretend it's lunchtime and you've stopped in a local restaurant. You have two choices: liver with brown rice sprinkled with brewer's yeast and steamed spinach, or a burger, fries, and Coke. Which would you choose? If you picked the burger lunch you're like many Americans. And like many Americans, you may not be getting enough B vitamins in your diet.

Here in the U.S.A. we have one of the best food supplies in the world. At any time of day or night we can select from thousands of food items. But in the absence of nutritional knowledge, too many choices can be a problem too. We can afford to be frivolous, so we often buy food for pleasure, not nutrition. We eat almost as a recreational sport. One result is overweight. A significant number of Americans lug around more fat than their bodies were built to carry.

But a more insidious result is borderline vitamin deficiencies, most notoriously of B vitamins. True, no one is walking around with pellagra. But many Americans place their health on a tightrope every day by barely meeting their minimum vitamin needs. Thiamin intake, for example, runs fairly close to the minimum. A fast-food meal of a hamburger, fries, and shake provides a large percentage of a day's calorie requirements but only 15 percent of the necessary daily nutrients. Fast foods and processed foods, because of their preponderance of refined ingredients, fats, and sugars, as well as their high cooking temperatures, won't fill the bill for the Bs.

We also put our health on the line when we consume excess alcohol. Even if our bodies had enough vitamins before we drank, we might be deficient by the time we'd sobered up. Alcohol requires B vitamins to break it down. But today's alcoholic beverages, unlike the mead (and the vitamin-rich beer) of yore, contribute no B vitamins to the body's pool. It uses up the body's B vitamins without contributing any in return.

Survey after survey finds that the intake of B vitamins is inadequate for many Americans, especially women, teenagers, and the elderly. While these people may not have deficiency symptoms, they may not be living up to their potential in terms of energy and achievement.

To B or Not to B: Supplementation

Mead is hard to come by these days. So is B-rich beer. "There's always liver," you might be thinking at this point. True, but organ meats are a case of good news/bad news. The good, of course, is that they offer a wonderful array of B vitamins. The bad news is that they are loaded with cholesterol and fat, substances that most Americans need to cut down on, so they should be consumed sparingly.

Unless we break out of habits of fast food, snack food, and white wine-accompanied lunches, many of us should consider getting more Bs into our lives with supplements. If you choose a B supplement, be careful. Not all B supplements are created equal. Remember, the vitamins work as a balanced team. Some supplements split up the team. They supply some parts of the B complex but skimp on some that are equally necessary.

You may purchase a supplement that contains only one B vitamin, say B_6. You then take it in copious amounts. Since B is water soluble, your body will excrete the excess vitamin through your urine. But, when it eliminates the extra B_6, your body eliminates along with it other B vitamins, such as folic acid or B_{12}. The upshot is that you will have created an imbalance. You will have hampered the team's ability to perform as a team.

Taking a supplement to make sure you get all the B vitamins you need is a good idea. But don't defeat the purpose. Read the label and make sure the supplement provides each member of the B team.

Introduction to Minerals

ANTHONY ALBANESE, PH.D.

Minerals are 5 percent of body composition and serve as a foundation for body metabolism. With the disruption of normal mineral metabolism, there are severe and often dramatic physiological and psychological results. Minerals are the catalysts that help enzymes to do their work. They also form the structure on which the body is constructed and are essential to nerve and muscle functions. Supplied adequately in an otherwise balanced diet, they make possible, although they do not guarantee, a healthy, strong body. Their absence in the diet may result in disturbances resembling those caused by pathogenic agents.

Minerals fall into two groups: *macrominerals*, those needed in the diet at levels of 100 mg per day or more, and *microminerals*, those needed in amounts no higher than a few milligrams per day, also known as trace elements. Minerals classified as macrominerals include calcium, phosphorus, magnesium, sodium, potassium, and chloride. Among important microminerals are iron, copper, zinc, manganese, iodine, sulfur, cobalt, and chromium. Industrial treatment of various foods provides the opportunity both for gains and losses of these trace elements.

Although iron is classified as a trace element in terms of relative tissue content, its many essential life functions qualify it as a major nutrient. Iron-deficiency anemia ranks second only to protein malnutrition, including kwashiorkor, in the number of people affected.

The trace elements present in plants and animal species have complex functions which could not be well defined until some thirty years ago for lack of sensitive analytical methods. They often interact; for instance, copper catalyzes the use of iron in blood formation.

Let's remember that many minerals have a multitude of functions. As an example, calcium is essential for the clotting of blood, the action of certain enzymes, and the control of the delivery of important biological messages to cells, in addition to its more familiar function in building bones.

A high consumption of highly refined or fabricated foods may substantially reduce the intake of essential minerals, unless these foods are properly fortified. A varied diet from as many natural food sources as possible will probably meet our requirements for essential minerals, inorganic and organic.

Realizing the gaps in our knowledge of trace-element requirements, the best and only advice that can be given to assure adequate trace-element nutrition is to consume a varied, mixed diet rich in unrefined foods and to supplement it, if in doubt, with a balanced supplement.

7

CALCIUM, MAGNESIUM, AND PHOSPHORUS
Sustaining the Skeletal System

You don't drink milk? Neither do many Americans. Billions of people all over the world don't drink milk. But, in obtaining a regular supply of calcium, other cultures have some advantages that Americans generally lack. These differences make a bone-deep difference in the body's calcium balance.

Calcium is one of the most important minerals needed by the body in large quantities, and milk is one of the best calcium sources there is. But in most of the world milk presents some difficulties. Some nations simply can't spare enough land for grazing herds of cattle. For other nations, the problem is not keeping cattle but processing the milk. It's a health problem. They lack the technology to pasteurize milk, and unpasteurized milk breeds tuberculosis. Even if people in the Middle East and Asia could get pasteurized milk, they would have trouble digesting milk. We say they are "lactose intolerant" because their digestive systems lack sufficient amounts of the enzyme needed to break down a milk sugar called lactose. (A few of these populations have adapted by ingesting fermented milk products, which are lower in lactose.)

Many of these populations tend to be shorter in height than most Americans and Europeans, but they have well-formed, dense bones and don't seem plagued with osteoporosis the way we are. As many as nine out of ten older American women show some evidence of bone disease; yet it is virtually unheard of in Third World nations. Here may be some reasons why:

1. Many populations that maintain a healthy calcium balance without dairy products live in either tropical or semitropical climates. Lots of sunshine guarantees enough vitamin D for optimum absorption of the calcium they do get, as we learned in Chapter 3.

2. Meat is a luxury for many Third World nations. People are primarily vegetarians, which bodes well for the bones.

3. Carting around weight, even your own in walking or jogging, is good for the bones. When was the last time you lugged water from a well? Or toted produce to or from a village marketplace miles away? People living in societies where even a bicycle is a luxury do plenty of that.

4. Some cultures in which people never touch a drop of milk after infancy add calcium to their diets in ways that the average American would never dream of. Like eating white clay, which is calcium. Ingesting clay, of course, can have serious side effects, so don't do it. But in some African cultures people mix some into their meals, especially those prepared for pregnant women. Let's take a quick look at some other clever dietary methods to obtain calcium.

Limestone Tortillas, Anyone?

How often do you eat Chinese food? Maybe once every few weeks if you live in New York or San Francisco. Perhaps less often if you live in Omaha. But, if you lived in Beijing, you'd eat Chinese food every day. Many of your meals would probably be cooked in the Chinese sweet-and-sour method. Dishes prepared this way rely on vinegar for their pungent punch. But, more than providing mere tastebud tingling, vinegar actually gives the meal a calcium bonus. The vinegar is so acidic that it partially dissolves any meat bones used to flavor the sauce. Calcium from the bones thus becomes part of the meal.

Vietnamese cooking applies this same ingenious method for supplementing calcium otherwise lacking in the diet. After they eat the meat from a fish or chicken, the Vietnamese make a rich soup stock by cooking the bones for hours with water, vegetables, and rice to form a rich, thick liquid. What else do they add? Vinegar, of course.

In Formosa, calcium carbonate is added to rice during its milling.

Europeans also developed many traditions for foods that are rich in calcium. No one is better than the Italians at making low-fat, high-calcium cheeses part of a meal. Many dishes, even desserts, make extensive use of cheeses like mozzarella and ricotta. Grated parmesan and romano are tableside condiments just like salt and pepper. Throughout Europe, notably in France, meals invariably end with cheese and fruit.

South of our own border, Mexicans soak the corn that they use to make tortillas in lime water. In addition to processing the corn with lime water, a pinch of ground limestone is added to the tortilla itself. This practice dates back thousands of years. Mexicans eat tortillas with nearly every meal and are thus assured a reasonable intake of calcium.

Animal, Vegetable, or Mineral?

Minerals in the body were detected quite early—iron was found in the blood in 1747. But an understanding of their functions had to await a more sophisticated chemistry. Today we still use the term "mineral," coined in simpler times when scientists thought they could easily categorize all matter. Back then, a mineral was anything that was not animal or vegetable. Today we know minerals are part of both animals and vegetables. We used to think of all minerals as inert, like rocks. Today we know that's not accurate. Calcium, for example, is extremely active in the body.

The name "calcium" comes from the Latin *calx*, which means "lime." This is also the origin of the word "chalk." We come into contact with calcium daily as chalk, eggshell, seashell, bones, or limestone. All of these sources can fulfill the body's calcium needs, and, as we have seen, in other cultures they do just that.

Boning Up on Calcium

Human beings, as we said in Chapter 1, eat a little over a pound (about 500 grams) of food per day on a dry-weight basis. Nearly all of this food comes in the form of carbohydrates, fat, and protein, but a tiny bit, about three or four grams, ought to come from minerals.

Much of that three grams should consist of calcium, which is what nutritionists call a "macromineral." The body requires a total of about a dozen minerals, most in amounts so tiny that they are called "trace elements." Not so calcium.

The U.S. Food and Nutrition Board estimates our daily calcium needs, depending upon our age, at 800 to 1,000 milligrams. Some scientists believe we need 1,200 milligrams. That's an average of about a gram per day, equivalent to about a teaspoon of limestone. By comparison, we need only about 300 to 350 milligrams of magnesium, 60 milligrams of vitamin C, and 18 milligrams of iron. Some mineral requirements are so tiny that they're measured in micrograms, like that for selenium.

Why so much calcium? Calcium makes up from 1.5 to 2.2 percent of the human body. If you weigh 160 pounds, about 3 pounds of you is calcium. About 99 percent of this calcium forms the skeleton, the bones, and the teeth. A strong, well-developed skeleton fulfills a number of functions. It gives the body form; protects the brain, the heart, and other organs; and serves as an anchor for muscles that allow the body movement. Also, the bone marrow is the site of blood-cell formation. Well-calcified bones are less likely to break or fracture. The remaining 1 percent of the body's calcium circulates through the bloodstream. But don't underestimate it just because it's a mere 1 percent. It makes possible all our muscle contractions, including our heartbeat, the most important muscle contraction of them all. It helps transmit nerve impulses, it plays a role in hormone function, and it's essential to the clotting of the blood. In fact, this 1 percent is so crucial to life that the body transfers enough calcium from the bones to the blood if it can't get it from the diet. Remember, the body is a fantastic survival machine.

The Calcium Balancing Act

"Drink your milk," we were told as children. Good advice. Now that we're grownup, no one tells us to drink our milk anymore. Why? Well, everyone knows that children build new bone as they grow. But most people think that once you're grown your bones stay the same—like the steel beams in a skyscraper. Nothing could be further from the truth. Bones are as dynamic as any other structure in the body.

The cells in the body—except for brain cells—turn over. That is, old cells constantly die, new ones are formed. This process uses up some of the energy you take in from food. During childhood and adolescence rapid growth requires a rich supply of nutrients. Children need a growth "allowance."

In some parts of the body, cell turnover takes place more quickly than in other parts. For example, you have a completely new intestinal lining every few days. This remodeling goes on more slowly with bone cells, but it does happen. New cells are formed; calcium supplied by the diet is deposited in the bones. If you looked at bone through a microscope, you'd see that it's structured so that most of the mineral crystals are close to a blood vessel. This helps the exchange of minerals and nutrients between bone tissues and body fluids.

All calcium from food first gets absorbed into the bloodstream after the food is digested. But only one percent of the body's calcium supply is supposed to be in the blood, remember? When there's more, say after you digest a glass of milk, a hormone stimulates the mineralization of bone. The extra calcium is removed from the blood and deposited in bone.

Can you guess what happens when there's not enough calcium in the blood? Perhaps you haven't included any calcium sources in your diet. Another hormone stimulates removal of calcium from the bone back into the blood.

This is how the body maintains calcium balance. It's the same as if you kept a checking account with a constant balance of $1,000 and a savings account with $99,000. Any amount over $1,000 in the checking account automatically transfers into the savings account. But if the checking-account balance dips below $1,000, enough funds will automatically transfer from the savings account to make up the difference. That's okay in a pinch, but if you keep writing checks and make no deposits, you will eventually deplete your savings. This is what many Americans do to their bones. And it's not just a matter of not getting enough calcium. Other items in the diet compound the problem.

Protein: Tipping the Balance

Vegetarians have a point—excess protein increases calcium excretion. Meat, a powerful protein source, is especially guilty of this. Given the typical American mania for meat, we've got a problem.

Except in the United States, Argentina, Australia, and much of Europe, people eat meats in little bits if at all. Again Chinese cooking comes to mind, but many other cuisines bear this out as well. Indian curry, Italian spaghetti sauce, and Mexican burritos all use meat almost as a condiment to flavor vegetables and grains rather than as the center of attraction. Much of our society, on the other hand, provides the body with large hunks of meat almost every day. We've also abandoned the European tradition of finishing a meal with cheese, which could help offset calcium losses caused by meat.

In societies with lower protein intakes, people get by with less dietary calcium. Many people, especially Asians, seem to maintain an adequate calcium balance on as little as a few hundred milligrams per day. Actually, that's about as much calcium as some Americans get, in spite of our government's recommendations. The difference is that people in many other societies manage to utilize more fully whatever calcium their diets provide.

By contrast, it is well known that about 60 percent of our dietary calcium winds up flushed down the toilet. It never makes it to our bones. Other factors like lack of exercise and exposure to sunshine most likely are involved. But we do ourselves no favors with excessive meat consumption.

Magnesium

Calcium is not a solo performer in its balancing act. Like nearly all nutrients in the body, it's part of a team. The other players on calcium's team are magnesium and phosphorus. In order for these nutrients to perform well together the diet must supply each of them in adequate amounts. Milk does this beautifully. But we don't drink much milk, and many of the foods we like to eat are low in calcium and magnesium.

Centuries ago, an unknown Roman proclaimed the health benefits of "magnesia alba" (literally, white magnesium), the salts found at Magnesia in Greece. These salts, he said, could cure all kinds of ailments. Others found this to be so, and people from all over the Roman empire flocked to Magnesia for the therapeutic salts. If they were suffering from deficiency of magnesium the symptoms would soon disappear. This was the first recognition of magnesium as a nutrient, and from this ancient spa the mineral got its name.

A similar phenomenon occurred in 1618 in a village south of London called Epsom. The village water supply was found to have wound-healing properties and a laxative effect. The substance formed after evaporation of the water was called "Epsom salts" (magnesium sulfate).

The RDA of 300 to 350 milligrams for silvery white magnesium is 20 to 25 percent greater than what we actually require. That's because this mineral is very difficult for the body to absorb.

In the technological world, magnesium is a light structural metal used in airplanes and tools. In the biological realm it's a central component of chlorophyll, the green pigment that enables plants to transform carbon dioxide and water into life-giving carbohydrates. Magnesium is also a major component of sea water, in which chlorophyll evolved.

The human body contains 20 to 28 grams of magnesium, more than half of it within the complex compounds we call bone. Magnesium is required for the maintenance of bone structure.

The remainder circulates throughout the body, for it is an important activator of enzymes, especially of those involved in energy. Here it works together with the B vitamins. Magnesium is also required for protein synthesis, the transmission of nerve impulses, and muscle contractions.

Magnesium deficiency can cause weakness, muscle cramps, vertigo, twitching, convulsions, and muscle rigidity—all of which indicate its role in the neuromuscular system. Behavioral disturbances such as depression, apathy, or delirium may also occur.

Although 60 to 70 percent of consumed magnesium is not absorbed, most Americans seem to get at least a bare minimum. In our society, clinical magnesium deficiency can occur, usually from malabsorption, diabetes, protein deficiency, chronic diarrhea, alcoholism, prolonged use of diuretics, or gross malnutrition. Deficiency that comes to the attention of a physician can be easily cured. Borderline deficiency is sometimes found among adolescents and college students. Athletes, because of increased losses through perspiration, may also be at risk.

As one might guess, plant products, whole grains, beans, nuts, and vegetables provide the richest magnesium sources, but processing these foods causes great losses. There is little magnesium left in rice and white flour, and none in sugar, fat, or alcohol.

Phosphorus

Calcium and phosphorus together make up about three-fourths of the mineral content of the body. The amount of calcium present is twice that of phosphorus. A full 80 percent of the body's phosphorus interlocks with the bulk of the body's calcium in the bones and teeth. The remaining 20 percent circulates to every cell via the bloodstream, for phosphorus takes part in all energy-yielding reactions.

Phosphorus abounds in our diets. Meats, poultry, and fish furnish fifteen to twenty times as much phosphorus as calcium (milk, cheeses, and green leafy vegetables are among the few foods that provide less phosphorus than calcium).

Meat, poultry, and fish are not the only popular American

menu items that increase our phosphorus intakes. Soft drinks now take first place as America's favorite beverage, far outdistancing milk in all marketing surveys. This is a relatively recent marketing phenomenon. Only 50 years ago, soft drinks were a novelty; a special treat. Back then, this newfangled drink was frequently called by one of its chief ingredients—phosphorus. "I'm going to the drugstore for a cherry phosphate," Grandpa might have said on occasion. He maybe had one a month. Now most of us drink two soft drinks a day.

The effect of dietary phosphorus on calcium balance is still under investigation. Animal studies have shown that excess is not favorable to calcium absorption.

The Fat Factor

There's more. At least one other nutrient excess in the American diet contributes to a calcium crisis—fat. Excess dietary fat can bind calcium into insoluble "soaps" that are excreted. Again we can point an accusing finger at meat because of its high fat content. Societies that do well on very little calcium are primarily vegetarian and hold their fat intake to 20 percent of their calories.

So the next time you think you deserve a fast-food break, think of your bones. If you must have that burger and large soft drink, try to make sure you get ample calcium too. Or your bones will eventually give you the kind of break you don't want: the broken bones of osteoporosis.

Osteoporosis: A National Epidemic

Osteoporosis is becoming one of the most important health problems in our population. This crippling bone disease afflicts some 20 million people in the United States, most of them elderly women. Osteoporosis can disable and perhaps even shorten the lives of elderly people. Hunched spines, loss of teeth, broken hips, and other fractures result from this deterioration of the bones. It's estimated that 90 percent of all fractures in people over 60 are due to osteoporosis.

Each year complications from hip fractures eventually kill

15 to 30 percent of all victims. Of those who survive, most are disabled and require nursing-home care. Experts estimate the cost of osteoporosis in this country at $3.8 billion annually.

Some loss of bone density occurs with age in just about everybody. But not everybody gets osteoporosis. The stronger the bones you've built throughout your life, the less likely you are to be incapacitated by losing a little bit. In fact, blacks, who genetically have strong bones, seldom get osteoporosis at all.

Diet appears to play a role in the development of this condition. A low calcium intake for most of one's adult years—a problem for most women—is thought by many authorities to be a contributing factor in osteoporosis.

The typical osteoporosis victim is a thin, elderly white woman whose lifelong calcium intake has been marginal. To paraphrase the old saying, the bone losses of old age so weaken the camel's back that it may break even without a straw being added.

Because of the hormonal change, bone loss accelerates after menopause, one reason why women are more susceptible than men. But the trouble starts in adolescence when kids switch from milk to soft drinks. For girls the situation is a bleak one, even without the fate their hormones have in store for them.

While fashions and pop stars are teenage girls' passions, looking stylishly thin is their obsession. Instead of exercising and eating a balanced diet—the real key to good looks—they crash-diet and drink gallons of diet soda. They frown on milk as "fattening" at a time when their bodies are trying to build adult-size bones.

In contrast, boys at this age are more likely to play active sports, and they haven't dropped milk entirely, thus adding to the bone mass that will carry into old age.

As girls grow up, the calcium crisis increases. On any day it is estimated that as many as 75 percent of all women do not consume the recommended 800 milligrams of calcium. A full 25 percent consume less than 300 milligrams. Soft-drink and meat consumption remain high.

Little by little, the body taps into the skeleton's calcium supplies. Some women already show a reduction in bone mass as early as age twenty-five and most show some decrease by thirty-five to forty.

The calcium demands of pregnancy and lactation can further "drain" bone mass. If the mother's intake isn't enough to meet both her needs and the child's, nature will see to it that the child is provided for. (We will discuss the nutritional costs of pregnancy further in Chapter 10.)

Also, the degeneration of the jaw bone is a primary reason why so many elderly people lose their teeth. Then once their natural teeth are gone, many older people can no longer eat fresh fruits and vegetables. Poor diet contributes to other health problems, especially in this vulnerable stage of life.

Trabecula bone also surrenders its calcium easily. This is the bone that makes up the vertebrae of the spinal column. By the time most women and some men are in their forties, they begin to experience occasional low back pain. Nearly all will attribute it to bad posture, a particular chair, their job, or middle age. Very few realize it may be a warning sign that the spine is weakening. If you were to examine the vertebrae in some of these people you'd see that the bone has started to give way and sag in the middle. But this is just one possible cause of low back pain. The problem could be a muscle sprain, kidney disease, or some other condition. Your doctor can help you determine what the matter is and whether osteoporosis may be a factor.

A woman's total bone mass at age eighty may be only half of what it was at forty. Much of the calcium that makes up the bone structure has been lost from the bone, released into circulation, and quickly excreted without ever being replaced. After being mined repeatedly, the bones are weak, brittle, and full of tiny holes like a dried-out old sponge—hence the name osteoporosis, "osteo" meaning "bone" and "porosis" meaning "porous;" literally "porous bones."

Thus weakened, the spine may no longer be able to support the body's weight. The vertebrae collapse on each other and the spine curves into a hunched back deformity known as "dowager's hump." Without the support of the spine, the weight of the shoulders shifts forward, creating a stooped posture. The abdomen is also pushed forward as the spine shrinks.

As a result of stooping over and having compressed vertebrae, the osteoporosis sufferer loses height, anywhere from two to six inches and sometimes more. She has become the stereotypical "little old lady." Although we once thought it was inevitable, now we realize this disfigurement may be preventable. But for many people the realization comes too late.

Because weakened bones can no longer properly support the body's weight, spontaneous fractures may occur. We used to think elderly women fell and broke their hips. Now we know that sometimes hips break first, then the women fall. But the slightest fall can cause any osteoporotic bone to break. And it's not a clean break as in a healthy bone. Brittle osteoporotic bones shatter like glass, spreading bits and pieces into the tissue. Resetting the bone usually requires a skilled orthopedic surgeon, who may have to use devices to hold the bone together, such as steel pins or prosthetic joints.

Osteoporosis may be stopped or even reversed. Calcium supplementation, estrogen therapy, and exercise have all been shown to increase bone density in the elderly. Fluoride treatment can slow but not reverse loss of bone density.

The total daily calcium intake required to maintain healthy bone density and calcium balance in postmenopausal women is now believed to be 1,000 to 1,500 milligrams. This is higher than the current RDA and much higher than the calcium intake of most older women. Bone-disease experts recommend that all menopausal women take calcium supplements if their diets lack this level of calcium.

Exercise and Bone Density: Use It or Lose It

This may come as a surprise to you, but physical activity influences bone health. Extensive studies on astronauts and bedridden hospital patients all pinpoint inactivity as a chief culprit in bone loss. The pull of muscle against bone during exercise actually helps stimulate bone cells to reproduce. Thus activity spurs bone renewal and helps calcium retention.

Weight-bearing exercise seems to be especially beneficial in maintaining bone mass. Gravity, it turns out, must play a role in this interaction. The body must pull its own weight against gravity to reap the greatest bone benefits.

Try to recall for a moment all those *National Geographic* photographs of people in nations where osteoporosis is not a problem. Visualize Egyptians carrying baskets and crockery full of grains or water balanced on their heads, or Chinese with wooden yokes across their shoulders from which hang buckets of water or rice. Weight-bearing exercise is a way of life in other parts of the world.

In the U.S., lack of exercise becomes part of a vicious circle. Many of us no longer have to strain to open the garage door. We don't even have to leave the easy chair to change television channels. To get our food, we need do nothing more arduous than wheel a supermarket cart down the aisles. In fact, our way of life does not demand that we do any exercise at all, and many of us don't—although we may wear jogging suits to the supermarket.

The damage to our bones from lack of exercise compounds the dietary deficiencies that erode bones little by little over the years. Once osteoporosis sets in, Grandma or Uncle Fred become even less active because the back hurts. This only makes the problem worse. The skeletal system was designed not for easy chairs but for action.

Studies comparing runners to nonrunners, active and inactive college students, Norwegian lumberjacks and Norwegians who are not lumberjacks all find that, given similar calcium intakes, the more active people have better bone density.

Even in the aged, bones respond positively to exercise. In one study, the average age of subjects was eighty-two. Light to moderate exercise caused a 4.2 percent bone increase over thirty-six months, while the nonexercising group experienced a 2.5 percent decrease. So use it before you lose it.

Kidney Stones and Bone Spurs

No discussion of calcium would be complete without attention to these two conditions. Just because you have either condition does not mean you should deprive your body of its fair share of calcium.

Kidney stones are caused by multiple factors, including heredity and diet. Even with kidney stones, you still need to take care of your body's calcium needs. Obviously someone prone to kidney stones should be under a physician's care; the patient should discuss his or her calcium needs with the physician.

Another misconception is that calcium intake leads to bone spurs or calcium deposits. Most researchers have found that these formations occur because of hormonal imbalances, and although they contain calcium, they are not caused by calcium intake.

A New Theory: Calcium and High Blood Pressure

There is much controversy in the scientific community concerning the possible role of low dietary calcium in the development of high blood pressure. Dr. David McCarron has advanced the hypothesis that in some people with high blood pressure a low calcium intake is one of the factors involved. For many people with high blood pressure, though, the evidence still points to too much sodium. (See Chapter 11, Sodium and Potassium: The Critical Balance.)

Calcium Supplementation

The use of lime in preparing tortillas and the vinegar and bones in Vietnamese soup stock didn't become overnight culinary sensations in their respective cultures. Over countless generations people came to believe that their children developed healthier bones, lived longer, and were stronger if they followed these particular dietary practices. They didn't know what calcium was, but without realizing it they were supplementing their diets with this important mineral.

Today we know approximately how much calcium we need and we know what foods contain it: dairy products, bones (in stews, soups, and canned fish), and leafy green vegetables. Yet the typical American meal pattern of bread and butter, meat and potatoes, salad or fruit, soft drinks or alcohol, coffee with non-dairy creamer, and dessert does not supply our needs. In fact, it may even increase them. Our body's calcium balancing system just wasn't designed to cope with the protein and possibly phosphorus excesses of the American diet. The solution then is simple. We should consume more high-calcium foods or, as in those other cultures, supplement our diets with calcium in some way.

8

IRON

The Red-Blood-Cell Mineral

A young woman makes her way through a public garden. She feels so tired that she sits on a bench to rest. Rummaging through her purse, she finds a mirror. Her cheeks and lips look pale, so she applies more lipstick and rouge. In a few minutes, when she feels rested, she will go on. This woman is not aware of it, but she may have iron-deficiency anemia. Yet iron is one of the most abundant elements on earth: the cast-iron bench on which she is resting contains more than she will need for the rest of her life.

The earth's crust is 5 percent iron, yet iron deficiency is the most prevalent nutrition disorder in North America. Anywhere from 15 to 25 percent of the population lack adequate iron.

Swords, Nails, and Popeye

Thousands of years ago, in the days of ancient Greece, Jason and his Argonauts sailed in search of the fabled Golden Fleece. Legend has it that, to augment their daring and strength, these adventurers would drink red wine mixed with filings from the sharpening of their swords. They thought it was their weapons' savage power that lent their drink its strength. But actually, in the acidic resinous grape wine, the sword filings dissolved. The real secret of the Argonauts' potion was that it was an effective iron supplement.

Consuming enough iron has always been a problem for people and sometimes, like Jason, they have found imaginative ways to solve it. During Europe's Middle Ages mothers would tell their pale and listless daughters to place a handful of nails into an apple, then a few hours later to withdraw the nails and eat the fruit. We know today that iron from the nails leached into the apples, providing a ready source of supplemental iron. The women just knew it returned the roses to their daughters' cheeks and put back the sparkle in their eyes. (Unfortunately, this method wouldn't work today. Nails are no longer always made of iron.)

In more recent times, during the cartoon animation heyday of the 1940s the character Popeye the Sailor emerged. If you remember Popeye, then you recall his love, Olive Oyl, and his arch rival Bluto. Poor Olive was forever being chased and abducted by Bluto. She'd holler to Popeye for help but he was often too lethargic and lacking in stamina to respond until he gulped down a can of spinach. "I'm strong to the finish 'cause I eats my spinach," he'd sing after subduing Bluto and rescuing Olive. Spinach is a rich plant source of iron.

Popeye it turns out was a modern incarnation of a long line of mythological figures created to encourage children to eat foods that are good for them. These figures always drew their strength from particular healthful foods. When examined, many of these myths evolved from people's need for iron.

Iron as the Carrier of Oxygen

How does iron make us mighty? How does it help keep us bright-eyed, rosy-cheeked, alert, and energetic? There's no magic involved, just biochemistry. Iron transports oxygen, the leader of nutrients. Moving through the bloodstream, iron in the form of hemoglobin picks up oxygen in the lungs and takes it to every cell in the body. Hemoglobin, part of all red-blood cells, contains a full 60 to 70 percent of the body's iron. Each molecule of hemoglobin can carry four molecules of oxygen. Iron is oxygen's faithful steed, its only carrier.

Cells rely on regular oxygen deliveries to help them derive the maximum amount of energy from the food we eat and from the fat our body burns in the absence of food. You could survive without water or food for several days, but go without oxygen for just a few minutes and the brain could suffer permanent damage; any longer could result in death.

If your body lacks adequate iron, you just won't have as much oxygen at your disposal. You won't be able to run as far or think as sharply. Not having enough iron prevents you from doing your best at anything because oxygen is such a key factor in everything we do.

Are You Anemic?

While you read the last three pages of this book your body, if it is normal, made about half a billion new red blood cells. But if your iron supply isn't up to par, the cells you made will be smaller, paler, and fewer than they ought to be. Like the anemic young woman in the beginning of the chapter, you too will look pale.

Red blood cells near the skin's surface make for the rosy cheeks long associated with glowing good health. Folk wisdom instructed prospective husbands to look for rosy cheeks and red lips as signs of good health when selecting a mate. To enhance their marriage prospects some women relied less upon sticking nails in apples than upon simply reddening their cheeks and lips with cosmetics. However, cosmetics only cover the pallor of iron-deficiency anemia; they can't cure the weakness and lassitude that come with it.

Without sufficient iron, the amount of work your muscles and other tissues are capable of handling will slip downhill. New evidence indicates that, in some cases, chronic iron deficiency can also cause insomnia. The brain, it seems, when deprived of its full oxygen supply, seeks to prevent the body from falling into the shallow breathing patterns of sleep. The heart has to work harder even in limited physical activity.

Your doctor can determine whether or not you are anemic by sending a small sample of your blood to a laboratory for analysis. The lab counts the number of red blood cells present in a smear made from the sample. Typical healthy red-blood-cell counts range from 4.5 to 6.3 million per cubic millimeter in males and 4.2 to 5.5 million in females. Be aware that you can be mildly iron deficient even if you have an adequate number of red blood cells that contain enough hemoglobin. Further blood tests may be needed.

Some of the body's iron is a constituent of myoglobin, a protein in muscle cells that provides a supply of oxygen for muscle metabolism. The body's second-largest concentration of iron is its reservoir in the liver, spleen, and bone marrow. These supplies may be depleted first without affecting hemoglobin. You may be low in emergency reserves and not even know it. Poor growth (in children), reduced physical fitness and work performance, lowered scholastic performance, reduced immunity to disease, digestive disturbances, and thin, brittle, or flattened fingernails can be symptoms of iron deficiency.

If iron deficiency becomes severe, all body functions eventually slow down and death ultimately results. This is unlikely for the average person, who, nonetheless, may be deprived of full vitality because of a borderline iron deficiency.

What You Get, What You Need

Iron plays hard to get. Very few foods provide substantial amounts. Foods that do provide iron can make it very difficult for the body to get at it. All kinds of biochemical barriers, especially in plant sources, can prevent absorption. Only 2 to 5 percent of the iron in vegetables, fruits, beans, and grains ever reaches the bloodstream.

Iron in meat has a better chance of making it; about 15 to 35 percent can be absorbed, provided it's not blocked by other components of a meal, such as the tannins in tea and coffee and the phosphates and carbonates that give our beloved soft drinks their fizz. The U.S. Food and Nutrition Board has tried to cope with all this in setting a recommended dietary allowance.

Iron is so crucial to our ability to use oxygen that the body recycles iron from old blood cells to new. Every day the body typically recycles 30 to 40 milligrams. The only way a substantial amount of iron leaves the body is through bleeding. Losses in urine, sweat, and sloughed-off skin, hair, and nail cells account for only one milligram per day (menstruating women pose a special situation we'll address below).

This one milligram is the basis for determining our minimum daily needs. To replace it, the iron recommendation for adult men, infants, children ages 4 to 10, and postmenopausal women is 10 milligrams per day, of which about a tenth is absorbed. Since rapid growth always requires extra iron, the recommendation for children 6 months to 3 years old is 15 milligrams and for teenagers it is 18 milligrams—the same as the requirement for women of childbearing age. That's not much. If you took a pinch of sugar from the bowl, you'd have more than 18 milligrams of it between your fingers. There are various good ways to get this much iron.

But children—or adults for that matter—seldom eat their spinach anymore. Nor liver. Nor blackstrap molasses. Nor anything made from honest-to-goodness whole-wheat flour. Together in one diet, these sources and others used to add up to enough iron.

To get 18 milligrams of iron the diet must provide at least 8 milligrams of iron for every 1,000 calories. But the diets of many people have become so diluted by processed foods that for every 1,000 calories we now average only about 6 milligrams of iron. No wonder that, according to nutrition surveys, nearly 60 percent of us don't get enough iron. Women, children, and teenagers have the biggest gaps between their iron needs and actual intakes.

A Special Problem for Women

Iron deficiency occurs for three basic reasons: lack of iron in the diet, poor absorption of the iron we eat, and loss of blood. The first two are everybody's problem. But loss of blood is mainly a woman's problem, except for bleeding ulcers or some other kind of internal hemorrhage. People with these medical conditions are (or, if they're not, should be) on diets carefully monitored by a doctor. But most healthy menstruating women are on their own when it comes to nutrition.

From infancy up to adolescence boys and girls share identical needs. But, once hormonal changes occur, their nutritional paths diverge, not to meet again until the last leg of life's journey —old age.

For iron, the divergence occurs around age nineteen. Once a young man has built all the blood cells and new muscle tissue for his adult body, his iron needs drop from the adolescent high of 18 milligrams daily to a maintenance level of 10 milligrams. And there he stays for the rest of his life.

However, for women it's another story. Once menstruation begins, iron needs remain at a high of 18 milligrams per day from puberty until menopause. A woman's diet must replace the iron she loses every month in menstrual blood. If her intake does not balance out her losses, a deficiency develops.

As in the case of calcium, so in the case of iron: women need more but consume less, and they pay dearly for the deficiency. The results may not be as overt as the broken bones of osteoporosis but they are perhaps more insidious. Fatigue, lack of stamina, and lowered immunity to disease can stand in the way of a woman's achieving her personal and professional goals. It's difficult to go to law school at night, be a Girl Scout Leader, or run a ten-minute mile if you're always pooped.

Most women in the United States live on 1,500 to 2,000 calories a day. If the average American diet provides only 6 milligrams of iron per 1,000 calories, then American women wind up with only 9 to 12 milligrams of iron daily, instead of the optimal 18.

Yet most women find it difficult to maintain their ideal weight even at these low calorie levels. The reason? Not enough exercise and too many calories from such treats as chocolate-chip cookies and potato chips. As iron-poor junk foods predominate in the diet, women may become iron deficient and too tired to exercise. Without enough activity to burn all the calories they eat, they put on weight, in response to which they eat even less and further reduce their intake of iron.

Think about it for a moment. Just to wash dishes a woman once had to chop trees for firewood, fetch water from a well or pump, build a fire to heat the water and then wash dishes

—after churning butter, kneading bread dough, and hand washing clothes. Today dishes and laundry are loaded in their respective washing machines, bread and butter are picked up at the supermarket.

All these modern conveniences save time but unfortunately also reduce the occasions for exercise. In order not to become overweight, women have adjusted their food intakes downward. (Men have too, but because of their larger size they still consume more than 2,000 calories per day as compared to 1,500 or so for many women.) Even if women ate twice as much as they do, however, they might still be deficient in iron unless they ate the right foods. Studies analyzing the diets of the 1984 U.S. Olympic ski teams found that female skiers, although they consumed nearly 3,000 calories a day, did not always get 18 milligrams of iron. They ate too many "empty calories"—foods that provided calories but few vitamins and minerals.

When women whose iron intakes are marginal become pregnant, disaster looms because nature gives the baby priority for all nutrients. Iron is needed to build the placenta as well as the unborn child's blood cells, muscle, enzyme systems, and other organs, such as the spleen and liver. The infant may be born with a healthy iron supply at the cost of the mother's own. I believe morning sickness is actually a nausea caused by lack of oxygen similar to high-altitude sickness. The difference is that in morning sickness oxygen is available to the lungs; there's just not enough hemoglobin to transport it to the cells. Taking an iron supplement will not "cure" morning sickness. Supplemental iron cannot accelerate the speed with which the body can make red blood cells; it can only help provide the raw materials to do so. Morning sickness is perfectly natural and will disappear when the mother's red-blood-cell supply catches up.

The baby's iron needs are enormous during those first few months, and the mother may not have enough for two. Many obstetricians now include iron in a prenatal supplement program. In fact, iron is such a problem for today's American woman that the U.S. Food and Nutrition Board recommends that *all* pregnant and lactating women take an iron supplement.

Eating Natural Foods

Let's go back now to the anemic young woman who opened this chapter. Let's say she realizes that she's tired and pale because she needs more iron. "How do I get it?" she wonders.

First of all, she could try eating more natural foods. Minerals may be lost in processing. Iron-deficiency anemia has become increasingly common as foods we eat are more and more refined. For example, milling cereals can remove 75 percent of the iron content from the grain.

Second, she could increase her ability to absorb iron by adding vitamin C to the meal. For example, the absorption of iron from corn, rice, and beans, normally poor, improves when they are consumed with sufficient vitamin C.

Third, unless she is a vegetarian, this woman could consider eating certain meats that contain far more iron than grains or vegetables do. At best, a half cup of cooked spinach provides only 2 milligrams of iron and kale provides only 0.7 milligram. A slice of whole-wheat bread provides 0.8 milligram. Remember, a woman of child-bearing age needs 18 milligrams per day. That's 13 cups of cooked kale or over 22 slices of whole-wheat bread. Of course many other plant sources, like beans, can provide small amounts too and it all adds up. But there's no denying it: meat is the best food source of iron.

Since animals, like us, need a certain amount of iron to live, meat provides a richer source of iron. Not all meat contains equal amounts: Much depends on how the animal was reared and slaughtered. Our food supply has changed greatly in the last twenty years or so. Now much of the iron-containing blood is removed from meat and sold for use in by-products.

Still, a large hamburger provides three grams of iron, a little better than spinach. It's downhill from there, though, with rib roast, chicken, and fish all providing one to two grams per serving.

The secret is a particular kind of meat—the liver. Time was when the butcher threw in a slice of liver for every piece of meat you bought. In those days families ate liver once or twice a week. Liver is the body's iron supply depot and that goes for animals, too. A slice of calf liver contains 12 milligrams of iron. Pork liver provides 24 milligrams. One drawback is that liver carries a heavy price tag in terms of cholesterol.

Another factor reducing iron intake is that we no longer cook in old-fashioned cast-iron pots and pans. These actually add significant quantities of iron to the foods cooked in them. But today we prefer color-coordinated enamel, aluminum, or nonstick coated cookware.

So if the young woman upped her caloric intake and ate several cups of cooked leafy green vegetables a day, one serving of liver, lots of beans and whole grains, with vitamin C, and cooked it all in cast-iron pots and drank no coffee with her meals, she might be able to rev up her system with the iron she needs.

She might be able to eat like this but can you? It doesn't hurt to try, but remember, a supplement with both iron and vitamin C can provide nutritional insurance in case your diet falls short of your intentions.

9

TRACE MINERALS

A Little Goes a Long Way

A man in New Jersey loses his ability to taste and smell. A woman in China has hands crippled with painful swollen joints resembling rheumatoid arthritis. A child on the island of Crete is born mentally and developmentally disabled. What do these afflicted people have in common?

Each is deficient in an essential mineral needed by the human body in minute amounts. The amounts are so small, in fact, that early biochemists working without today's advanced techniques could barely discern them in tissue samples. Hence the biochemists called them trace minerals.

Our requirements for trace minerals range from milligram amounts for iron and zinc down to micrograms for minerals more recently discovered in the body, such as selenium and chromium. In the body, the total of *all* trace elements is 25 to 30 grams, about one ounce, compared to over 1,000 grams of calcium and about 30 grams of magnesium.

Trace minerals are among the pieces most recently fitted into the human nutrition puzzle. The essential functions of some were discovered as recently as the 1960s and '70s. For some of these trace minerals not enough is known yet for the government to establish a recommended daily allowance specific for age and sex. That refinement awaits future decades. However, scientific understanding of some trace elements has enabled the government to at least set "safe and adequate ranges" for them. We will look at these trace elements and at zinc in this chapter.

Blue-Flour Tortillas

As Mexican food becomes more popular in the United States, most of us are within driving distance of a Mexican restaurant. There we might savor tortillas, a chewy, crêpe-like pancake made from corn flour. Ours would be served to us light golden brown the way gringos like them. But, in the southwestern part of the country, people of Mexican extraction prepare "blue-flour" tortillas, following the custom from south of the border.

A blue-flour tortilla starts out like any other tortilla, but before cooking it, a Mexican dusts each side with ashes. When the tortilla is cooked, the ash gives it the bluish tinge.

Why, I wondered when traveling in the Southwest, would people with a limited diet purposely make a staple food look less appealing? As we have seen in preceding chapters, food patterns are influenced by such factors as scarcity, religious customs, and nutritional advantage. As a nutritionist, I had a hunch that the ash on the tortilla contributed to good health.

Recall that tortillas are made from corn kernels. In subsistence societies such as those of the Native Americans and native Mexicans, nothing is wasted. The corn cobs are used as miniature fuel logs to boil water and cook. Meanwhile the leaves, stems, and stalks of the corn plant are reduced to the ash that I believe is the Mexican family's trace-mineral supplement. The ash contains the minerals the corn plant absorbed from the soil. These include calcium, iron, and other elements, ranging from zinc to copper. The blue cast of the tortilla comes primarily from oxidized copper (think of the color of an old copper kettle). In addition to the ash, the Mexican mother also adds limestone to her tortilla flour, which provides her family with calcium and magnesium.

Iodine: Seaweed and Burnt Sponge

Today, calling someone a cretin is just another insult implying stupidity. But the term derives from a specific form of mental retardation called cretinism. This was a tragedy that befell children born long ago on the island of Crete, where iodine-deficient soil prevails. Cretinous children have underdeveloped thyroid glands. They live short life spans as mentally disabled, partially deaf dwarfs.

In adults, this iodine deficiency manifests as goiter, a grotesque swelling of the neck. If unattended in its early stages, a goiter will continue to grow. Eventually it can become large enough literally to choke the iodine-deficient individual to death.

Goiter was known in China as early as 3000 B.C. and has afflicted people all over the world. One of the saddest aspects of iodine deficiency, whether it is seen as cretinism in newborns or as goiter in adults, is that prevention or cure is so simple.

If all the other nutrients involved in metabolism are thought of as a vast symphony orchestra, iodine is the conductor. It operates by forming two key hormones in the thyroid gland, thyroxine and triiodothyronine, which together are keys in the regulation of metabolism. These hormones are required for growth, reproduction, nerve formation, and mental health, bone formation, protein synthesis, and all aspects of energy metabolism. Without iodine in the diet none of these activities can take place properly.

Our RDA for iodine is only 150 micrograms (more for pregnant and lactating women). This is so small an amount that the weight of iodine an adult woman requires for a whole year would amount to only three days of her iron requirement. The government has set the RDA at double our minimal needs to provide a margin of safety.

Unfortunately for people and animals, plants don't require iodine for growth. So, unlike other minerals, iodine is present in plants only if they happen to grow in iodine-rich soil.

When there's not enough iodine in the diet, the whole system just slows down. The person becomes listless and inactive. As the thyroid gland strains to catch any bit of iodine the blood might contain, it swells. The swelling increases to form the goiter.

Interestingly, the sea abounds with iodine. In many cultures where goiter and cretinism may have been endemic at one time, someone no doubt noticed that those who ingested ample seafood and sea plants thrived. Thousands of years ago, the Chinese effectively treated goiter by feeding seaweed or burnt sponge to the stricken. In fact, because the same methods were used by the Incas of Peru, some anthropologists theorize that the Incas are descendants of the same people. Greek and Egyptian fishermen also consumed the ash from burnt sponge to avoid the symptoms of iodine deficiency. Today dried seaweed, shellfish, and other types of seafood continue to be principal sources of iodine for many cultures.

In the United States, iodine deficiency is a thing of the past. In 1918, when men drafted for World War I were examined, it was discovered that goiter was a problem only in certain low-iodine regions such as the Great Lakes states and the Pacific Northwest. Scientists further realized that farm animals from goiterous regions also suffered from deficiency symptoms. Many studies were done, and by the 1920s it became clear that simply iodizing common table salt would solve the problem. Also, our modern food-distribution system ensures that no one is dependent solely on locally grown produce. Thus we have eliminated the "goiter belts" in this country.

In fact, because of our increased intake of salt-processed foods as well as iodine's use in animal feed and food additives, our intakes have skyrocketed in the last few decades. A typical fast-food meal of a burger, fries, and a shake provides three times the RDA. Some scientists fear we may even be approaching toxicity levels.

A word of caution here. Because of its crucial metabolic role, iodine sometimes becomes part of weight-loss fads. A few years back, a diet book appeared that featured vitamin B_6, iodine-containing kelp, and vinegar. Since the B vitamins and iodine play essential metabolic roles, people were led to believe that ingesting extra B_6 and iodine would accelerate metabolism and burn calories faster. The vinegar was supposed to help dissolve the fat. None of this is true. Fortunately for the author, the diet plan contained only 1,000 calories per day, so people who followed it did indeed lose weight.

Selenium: Tea and Locoweed

About two thousand years ago in parts of China, people learned to brew a tea from a plant called astragalus. The tea wasn't a refreshment; it was medicine. Drinking the tea prevented or cured Kashin-Bek disease, which caused swollen joints and complete disintegration of cartilage.

Kashin-Bek disease is a sign of selenium deficiency. China's soil, even today, has the world's lowest selenium levels. Plants of the genus Astragalus are known throughout the world as selenium-accumulator plants. They can extract any bit of available selenium from the soil. In fact, where soil selenium levels are high, the plants accumulate so much that they become toxic. In the western parts of the United States, for example, a type of this plant is called locoweed because when grazing livestock consume it they develop a disorder known as "blind staggers" and eventually die. Yet in parts of China the soil is so poor in selenium that similar plants supply just enough selenium to meet people's needs.

But China is a vast nation with a billion people and unfortunately not all of them were aware of, or had access to, astragalus tea. In 1979, after millennia of intensive agriculture, the selenium in some rural areas was so depleted that epidemic numbers of local people—especially children and women of child-bearing age—began to develop deficiency diseases. The situation was desperate and the Chinese government turned to scientists all over the world for help. In fact, I was present when another scientist showed a physician an x-ray of a Chinese child's hand. "My gosh, it's a perfect case of rheumatoid arthritis," the doctor exclaimed. He was quite surprised when he found out it was Kashin-Bek disease. In addition, another disorder emerged— Keshan disease, which causes fatal deterioration of the heart muscles.

For a four-year period, the Chinese government fed nearly forty thousand children selenium orally and the death rate was greatly reduced. Many scientists diligently followed the proceedings since it would be impossible to induce similar conditions clinically on volunteers. Tragic as nationwide epidemics are, they have one silver lining. They usually help scientists discover something new and important about human health. This was just as true for selenium in 1979 as it was for niacin in the 1920s.

Selenium, scientists now know, works with vitamin E to help protect cell membranes from oxidative damage caused by harmful chemicals (see Chapter 4). Among these potentially harmful chemicals are the so-called free radicals or peroxides similar in action to the ones used in some laundry bleaches. Free radicals can be a result of natural events such as the cosmic rays that bombard our planet or of artificial conditions such as auto exhaust fumes and factory smoke.

In animals, lack of selenium weakens blood capillaries, causes muscular dystrophy, and damages hearts. Of these, only the heart problem has been found in selenium-deficient humans along with the arthritis-like Kashin-Bek disease.

It may be a coincidence that Americans living in states with high levels of soil selenium show lower death rates for some types of cancer than those in other states. But it is important to keep in mind that these people are not consuming excessive amounts of selenium, otherwise they would have a high death rate from selenium overdose. It can be an extremely toxic mineral in large doses.

Selenium intakes in the U.S. are sufficient to avoid serious deficiencies. Soil and water levels vary across the North American continent but the average American's selenium intake is believed to be 100 micrograms per day. The government's current safe and adequate range is set at 50 to 200 micrograms per day.

However, recent studies by Dr. Julian Spallholz showed that only 60 percent of ingested selenium is absorbed. This may indicate that, although American intakes may be sufficient to prevent deficiency diseases, they may be inadequate to provide the full benefit of selenium's antioxidant protection.

Seafood, meat, and whole grains can be good selenium sources. If you choose to supplement your diet with selenium, remember that a little bit goes a long way. The total selenium in your body would fit on a match head. As small an amount as 2.5 milligrams a day can be toxic to humans.

Copper: A Penny in the Pickle Jar

There's an old saying about putting a penny in the pickle jar. Pickles were homemade in the old days. Every homemaker wanted to put up pickles that the family would enjoy and that might win a ribbon at the county fair. The penny helped keep the pickles just the right shade of green. It was supposed to be healthy, too. And it was.

Copper is the element at work here. As the copper in the penny began to dissolve in the pickling solution, it turned blue-green, just as the copper in the corn ash turns the Mexicans' tortillas blue. Both the penny and the ash are a means of supplementing the diet with copper.

All plants require copper. In humans, copper helps the body produce the hemoglobin in red blood cells. It functions in many important enzyme reactions and thus also takes part in energy metabolism.

We don't need very much copper. The government's safe and adequate range is 2 to 3 milligrams per day. An adult body contains only 75 to 150 milligrams. This is less than you'd find in a penny. In fact, a penny probably contains enough copper to last someone a year.

As a rule we absorb nearly half the copper we consume. Interference by high levels of zinc in the diet or extensive use of antacids leaves us with less. Like magnesium, copper also is lost in perspiration. Some scientists argue that, when a person perspires profusely, say during heavy exercise or extreme heat, too much copper may be lost. This could be a health hazard for athletes.

Copper deficiencies, when they do occur, show up as pallor, convulsions, poor growth, scurvy-like sores, and prematurely gray hair. High doses of copper can relieve these symptoms but everyone with gray hair does not have a copper deficiency. Otherwise, people could just take copper supplements and no one would ever go gray.

Although copper deficiencies are rare so far, the processed foods that form an ever-increasing proportion of our diets are poor sources. Copper is present with other minerals in all natural foods. Some of the richest sources are organ meats, beans, shellfish, nuts, and cocoa. People may inadvertently get a copper boost from copper cooking utensils, water pipes, or the machinery used to pasteurize milk.

A well-balanced multivitamin-multimineral supplement can also ensure that intake is adequate. But copper bracelets, while possibly attractive jewelry, are worthless for copper supplementation or any other kind of disease "cure."

Without Zinc It Stinks

In the early 1970s a man who had a very profitable pizza parlor in New Jersey was disturbed when the pizza aroma he loved so much suddenly became disgusting to him. As days went by, the scent of his product became more and more obnoxious until he could no longer tolerate it. He sold his pizza parlor and tried to find another way to earn a living. But by then other familiar smells and tastes began to take on different characteristics, some distinctly nauseating. Doctor after doctor failed to find anything wrong.

Finally his case was referred to the National Institutes of Health. There, Dr. Richard Henkin identified the problem as zinc deficiency and treated it accordingly. Henkin named this disorder, wherein the ability to smell and taste becomes confused, "disgusia." Zinc deficiency may also be the culprit, he found, in a variation he called "agusia." In this form, the individual loses the ability to taste or smell anything.

These discoveries catapulted zinc into new prominence. Barely ten years had passed since zinc was found to be essential to human health. This discovery, in the 1960s, occurred when areas in the Middle East were found to have a high incidence of people with dwarfism and undeveloped sexual organs. In classic nutrition studies, young men with these disorders grew in stature and developed normal sexual characteristics after being provided with zinc supplements. (If zinc deficiency persists too long, however, it cannot be reversed: the individual must go through life without ever reaching full physical maturation.)

From these studies scientists concluded that zinc was essential to various types of metabolism and protein synthesis involved in growth and development. Thanks to the work of Henkin and others, we now also know that zinc is involved in literally dozens of enzymes, each vital for the growth and metabolism of certain cells and tissues. In fact, no other nutrient in the body is part of so many enzymes. There are only two grams of zinc in the entire body, but they really get around.

Zinc is one of the many nutrients necessary for the immune system. It may help prevent infection by its role in regulating the functions of some white blood cells. White blood cells are one of the body's important lines of defense against invading bacteria or viruses.

A preliminary study by Dr. George Eby indicates that very large amounts of zinc may help reduce the severity of a cold. Although the reason is not clear, it could be connected with zinc's role in the immune system. But such large amounts of zinc can cause other problems and should not be used to treat a cold without a doctor's guidance.

In cases of severe zinc deficiency, one of the symptoms is poor wound healing. This involves zinc's role, together with vitamin C, in the synthesis of protein, particularly of collagen, the protein that forms the skin's connective tissue. When a wound heals, the body has to make extra collagen and other proteins to replace what was lost. Without adequate zinc, this will naturally take much longer.

Zinc ointment has been found to help cuts heal. One may speculate that applying zinc to the damaged cells may help the body fight infection as well as repair the wound.

Zinc is also important to vitamin A metabolism. Zinc deficiency can lead to lower vitamin A levels in the blood, just as a deficiency of vitamin A itself would. Vitamin A is also responsible for the health of skin cells. Zinc's connection to vitamin A led scientists to investigate a possible role for zinc in relieving some skin conditions.

Zinc is now being studied experimentally in a number of conditions. These include alcohol-induced liver disease, surgery, burns, sickle cell disease, and cystic fibrosis.

The adult RDA for zinc is set at 15 milligrams. The body actually needs 2.5 to 4 milligrams per day but only 10 to 40 percent of the zinc we ingest is absorbed.

Although zinc is available in all plants and animals, zinc from animal sources is twice as well absorbed by the human body. The zinc in many plant sources is poorly absorbed because it is bound up with indigestible substances. Among plants the best sources include beans and whole grains; among meats the best are red meat, organ meat, oysters, and poultry. Often processing foods eliminates much of their zinc content, as it removes so many minerals, vitamins, and other nutrients.

Many Americans have cut down on meat to reduce cholesterol. Unless they increase their consumption of whole grains and beans, they may not get enough zinc. As with many other nutrients, anyone in our society who doesn't eat large quantities of nutritious food daily may also have a marginal zinc intake. Children, women, the elderly, and the poor usually fall into this category.

But the zinc picture may even be worse than that. New government research indicates that, given typical American food preferences, an intake of 3,400 calories would be required to obtain the 15 milligrams RDA for zinc. Unless you're a teenage boy or a hard-training athlete, it's unlikely that you eat anywhere near that much. Athletes may even need more zinc since it may be lost through sweat.

Another factor that can jeopardize the body's zinc supply is alcohol. So add alcoholics to the list of those apt to be zinc-deficient. This is especially harmful during pregnancy, for the fetus may be deficient in zinc.

Think you may not be getting enough zinc? A blood test is still the best way to find out for sure. Normal zinc levels in blood serum average about 100 to 120 micrograms per 100 milliliters. Below 80 micrograms is considered low. Be wary of hair analysis as an indicator—shampoos, bleaches, conditioners, and other environmental factors can all distort the results.

The Trouble with Too Much Zinc

Considering the magnitude and scope of zinc's role in the body, it may be prudent to supplement zinc in the diet up to the RDA level. But be sensible. The theory that "if a little is good, more is better" does not fit for zinc. Excess zinc can reduce absorption of copper. At ten times or more the RDA level, zinc can even interfere with the body's cholesterol balance, causing a shift toward the harmful kind of cholesterol that causes heart disease (see Chapter 12, on fats and oils).

The Zinc-Acne Controversy

In ancient days, some people believed that wiping a cloth across the face at the instant a shooting star passed through the sky was a cure for acne. In this case, the ancients were wrong. Many of today's topical creams and ointments aren't much better.

Acne, the agony of adolescents—and some adults—still remains somewhat a mystery. But researchers are narrowing the possible causes and cures. Minor evidence indicates that zinc may be involved.

Is it possible that the physical and emotional stresses of puberty combined with a marginal zinc deficiency manifest as acne? After all, the typical American teenage diet is known not to be optimal. The changes that occur in adolescence take place so rapidly they may outpace the body's ability to mobilize its zinc resources. Remember, though, acne is believed to have many causes. If a particular individual's acne is unrelated to zinc, taking supplementary zinc will not help.

Fluorine: The Cavity Fighter

Fluorine is another trace element with a fine line between not enough and too much. In the 1930s, residents of Arizona, Colorado, and the Texas panhandle were in a panic because their teeth were becoming mottled. Chalky spots appeared on the enamel and later turned an unsightly dark brown. What was the matter? Were they being poisoned?

The matter, it turned out, was abnormally high concentrations of fluorine in their drinking water. Although disfiguring, the mottled teeth were not a health threat. In fact, the teeth of children in these areas proved to be more resistant to tooth decay than those of children where the fluorine content was lower.

By the 1940s scientists had found an ideal level of fluorine that would prevent tooth decay without causing mottled teeth. Fluoridating public drinking water to that level, one part per million, is now a scientifically accepted, safe, economical public-health measure.

An adult body contains 2 to 3 grams of fluorine, primarily in bones and teeth. This fluorine needs to be replaced as cells turn over. The government's safe and adequate range of intake for most people is 1.5 to 4.0 milligrams. With fluoridated drinking water, that's about what we take in every day, although aluminum-containing antacids can interfere with fluorine absorption.

Toxicity from fluorine, called fluorosis, only occurs with intakes of 20 milligrams or more daily over long periods of time. This is about eight times the normal intake from food and fluoridated water. Severe tooth and bone deformities are the symptoms of fluorosis.

A more likely problem, particularly if you live in an area without fluoridated water, is not enough fluorine. Indisputable scientific evidence has found that fluorine is essential to the stability and strength of bones and teeth even though it is not one of the major structural components. Think of fluorine as being like the rubber taps the shoemaker puts on the heels and toes of your shoes to keep them from wearing down.

Fluorine is especially important for developing strong teeth that will last a lifetime. Therefore, it is crucial early in life. Teeth begin development during the tenth to twelfth week of pregnancy, and some studies have found that supplementing the diet of pregnant women with fluorine at that time produces offspring with virtually cavity-proof teeth. Many prenatal supplements now contain fluorine. Children who live in areas with unfluoridated drinking water now often have fluorine applied directly to their teeth by the dentist.

Fluorine may also be important in old age for treatment and prevention of osteoporosis. It cannot take the place of supplemental calcium or hormonal therapy in keeping bones strong, but it may help stop further erosion of calcium from the bones. Some scientists now suggest that a fluorine deficiency may be one of the causes of osteoporosis.

A rumor circulating some years back that fluorine caused cancer kept some communities from fluoridating their water supply. Although this allegation has no basis and has been refuted by the American Cancer Society and the National Cancer Institute, it continues to send many people to the dentist's chair.

Chromium: The Beer Mineral

When various cultures around the world learned to make beer, they were supplementing their diets not only with B vitamins (see Chapter 6), but with chromium. Although the B vitamins may be gone, beer drinkers, take cheer. Your favorite brew is still a good source of this trace mineral.

Imagine people's surprise back in the chrome-plated 1950s, when two U.S. scientists discovered that the shiny metal adorning bumpers and tail fins was actually required by the human body. The amount needed is small (.05 to .2 milligram) but vital to assist the hormone insulin in its action, which controls glucose metabolism. Although its exact chemical nature is still under study, chromium's active form is called the glucose tolerance factor (GTF).

The body contains very little chromium; about 6 milligrams, and this declines with age. When chromium is deficient, insulin function is impaired, and certain forms of diabetes may result. A slight deficiency that might be tolerated in a younger person, when combined with the natural losses of old age, is thought to cause some cases of adult-onset diabetes. But this type of diabetes caused by chromium deficiency is rare; most adult-onset diabetes cases are simply the result of overweight.

As in the case of selenium, the amount of chromium in foods depends greatly on the amount in the soil. Processing and refining reduce the chromium content of foods considerably. For example, white flour contains much less than whole wheat.

But don't rush out to buy a chromium supplement. It seems that the best way to obtain chromium containing the crucial GTF is from beef or pork kidneys, again indicating the nutritional power of organ meats, or from wheat germ or brewer's yeast. Besides, considering the infrequency of chromium deficiency symptoms in this country, it's apparent that a varied and well-balanced diet provides all we need.

Concepts in Health

WILLIAM HASKELL, PH.D.

The complexity of the life cycle, from birth to old age, is reflected in the changing needs of the human body. Before nutrition became a formal science, people realized that their needs for amount and type of food changed as life advanced.

The early years of life, pregnancy, lactation and very old age are extremely sensitive to nutritional deficiencies. The fast-growing infant and child need to build bone so rapidly that a vitamin D deficiency can soon result in bowed legs. A calcium-deficient diet can cause a pregnant woman to lose calcium from her bones, and the menstruating woman can easily develop an iron-deficiency anemia should she not consume enough iron-rich foods.

There is another side to the picture of poor nutrition: the excessive consumption of certain types of food over a lifetime. For instance, a diet too high in saturated fats and cholesterol could lead to diseases of the heart and blood vessels. Some minor changes may be valuable to help the body prevent these diseases: vegetable oils high in unsaturated fats have been recommended for some years to help in the prevention of some types of heart disease. Populations such as the Eskimos may have been protected by special fats contained in the fish they eat. Studies are in progress to see if these fats added to the American diet can help in preventing some heart and circulatory problems.

Certain types of adult diabetes may be caused by

overweight, while excessive consumption of salt in people with an inherited sensitivity can cause high blood pressure.

Occasionally, previously untested popular remedies have been found to contain some interesting compounds: for example, garlic has some factors that may affect blood coagulation in experimental conditions, but this evidence needs more testing in humans.

In regard to cancer, this most dreaded disease, is there a possibility that its prevention in certain situations may be connected with nutrition? Much more research is needed, and the answer is very complex. Perhaps some antioxidant vitamins such as E and C may play a role. Fiber has been found to be protective in animal experiments. Beta-carotene is a precursor of vitamin A that is also undergoing intense investigation in this regard. We do not have the answer yet, but certainly a nutritionally balanced diet can help to build resistance to many diseases. Let's remember that we are discussing prevention and not cure!

As we look over the human life cycle, there is no doubt that during periods of special stress—such as growth, pregnancy, lactation, and old age—one must be sure that all the vitamins and minerals are present in the diet in sufficient amounts. A supplement may be needed should the diet not ensure a sufficient intake.

IO

PREGNANCY

A Time of Special Needs

In Africa it was once common for pregnant women to eat nodules found around termite hills. The nodules, which form around the base and sides of these six- to ten-foot hills, are the fecal droppings of the termites. These insects ingest all kinds of natural materials, including plants, clay, and even dead animals. When the droppings were analyzed, they proved to be an excellent source of minerals—iron, calcium, magnesium, and others required by a pregnant woman. In fact, they compare favorably to a modern prenatal supplement.

It's not clear how the African women discovered the benefit of these termite nodules. In any case, the information was passed from one generation to another. Tribes whose territories were abundant with termite mounds would harvest the droppings and, using clay as a binder, press them into "eggs." When dried, these eggs would be sold to neighboring tribes whose territory was not so well endowed. This could have been the world's first supplementation industry.

Clay as a supplement can be traced to West Africa. The practice was transported to this country by slaves who continued to eat clay in their new environment for nutritional and cultural reasons.

The consumption of material that is strange but that often seems to satisfy a nutritional requirement is called "pica." For example, pregnant women who are anemic sometimes consume certain types of iron-rich clay which, it turns out, could provide the 30 to 60 milligrams of supplemental iron per day required. We know today that eating chalk, another form of pica among pregnant women, is one way of getting adequate calcium. Chalk is a form of calcium carbonate and it provides calcium for the bones of the infant and for the mother. Owing to toxic contaminants such as lead, pica can be quite dangerous, yet it is still common among poor undernourished women, even in this country.

Why are these mothers-to-be drawn to eating unpalatable substances such as chalk and clay?

In all living creatures, nature favors reproduction. From the instant a woman becomes pregnant until the birth of the child, everything in her body is reoriented toward producing a healthy child capable of thriving in our environment. As a result of this biological priority, women have been able to give birth under extreme conditions—conditions that in twentieth-century United States we would consider downright dangerous. Births occur in prison camps, among nomads living on the plains of the Gobi Desert, among natives in the jungles of Brazil, and among peasants on the rice paddies of China.

Hormonal changes in pregnancy lead to extraordinarily efficient use of nutrients, but unless the mother somehow gets all the nutrients needed by the fetus, the material will be "borrowed," when possible, from her own reserves. If calorie intake is insufficient and the mother has no fat reserve, the mother's own protein may be burned to supply the material the baby needs. Likewise, iron needed by new red blood cells can come from the mother's supply. Although nutrients can thus be provided from the mother's own tissues, she pays a cost in her health. That's why the African mothers eat clay or chalk, in order to supplement their normal intake of the minerals these materials contain.

Iron, calcium, and calorie intakes are problems for many women. Pregnancy can worsen any borderline deficiencies that may exist. For this reason teenage pregnancies can be especially hazardous, because young women are more likely to be on the nutritional brink. The result could be double tragedy: a deformed or retarded baby and a teenage girl with serious health consequences.

The Special Needs of Pregnancy

During pregnancy tremendous changes take place. A woman who gives birth to an average 7½-pound infant gains approximately 24 pounds. Of the other 16½ pounds, 4 represent the volume of blood that the mother must develop in order to supply the placenta and those organs that have become enlarged to support the developing infant. The placenta itself, which allows the nutrients to pass from the mother to the infant, will weigh one full pound. The mother's uterus and the muscles that support the uterus increase by 2½ pounds. The mother's breasts increase by 3 pounds. The fluid necessary to support the infant in the amniotic sac weighs 2 pounds. The mother puts on approximately 4 pounds of fat, which provides an energy source. This adds up to 24 pounds in a nine-month period.

To gain 24 pounds in a nine-month period requires an increase in caloric intake by approximately 15 percent or about 300 extra calories a day. Over a period of nine months, this comes to approximately 80,000 calories! Of these, about 50,000 calories are needed to create new maternal tissue and 30,000 calories to create the infant. Women who continue exercising and working and women carrying twins will have even greater energy needs.

What does it take to support the growth of a healthy fetus? There are many ways to translate those 80,000 calories into foods. I have selected examples to illustrate the energy needs of the mother for the baby, in addition to her regular diet. Items have been taken from the major food groups, and although complete in protein, fat, and carbohydrates, and with adequate fiber, the diet still lacks some vitamins and minerals that must be made up by supplementation. Fifteen to 20 percent of the calories come from protein, 30 percent from fat, and 50 to 55 percent from carbohydrates.

Remember: all this is on top of the mother's own normal needs.

In most cases the increased need for particular nutrients is greater than the increased calories can supply. Thus, food supplements are helpful. For example, although calorie needs increase only by 15 percent, the need for some of the B vitamins increases by 100 percent. One of these vitamins, folic acid, is required for red-blood-cell production (Chapter 6) and for cell division, including the reproduction of genetic material. It is indispensable. Needs for vitamins A, E, riboflavin, and B_6, and for iodine increase by 25 percent; for vitamin C, thiamin, B_{12}, and zinc by 33 percent; and for calcium, phosphorus, and magnesium by 50 percent.

Pregnancy has come a long way since the African woman was sent out to eat the droppings at the base of a termite mound. Now women can purchase prenatal supplements that usually provide most of the necessary vitamins and minerals, including folic acid, the vitamin of most concern during pregnancy. Two minerals that cannot be obtained in adequate amounts from most multivitamin prenatal supplements are calcium and magnesium, but, thanks to nutrition engineering, these can be easily obtained from a separate supplement. The mother-to-be must absorb approximately an extra 100 milligrams of calcium per day. It follows, owing to absorption inefficiencies, that she must take in approximately 400 extra milligrams of calcium daily during pregnancy.

Bones and teeth form and calcify during the latter half of fetal life and during the first few months after birth. This means that in the early part of pregnancy the mother must increase the density of her bones so that near the end of pregnancy and during lactation she can give some up as required by the developing child, without depleting her own skeleton.

Iodine requirements increase by 15 percent. Selenium needs increase also, and after the first three months, fluoride is required so the infant's teeth will be resistant to tooth decay. Although these trace elements do not yet have a specific RDA, they should not be ignored in a prenatal supplement program. Fluoride is very important during pregnancy, not necessarily for the mother, although it turns out that fluoride can help strengthen bones and may help women resist the ravages of

Additional Food Required by a Woman During the Nine Months of a Pregnancy

Food Group	Item	Amount
Milk	Milk	75 cups
	Yogurt	25 cups
Vegetables	Green peppers	3
	Eggplant	2
	Cucumbers	2
	Celery	½ bunch
	Cauliflower	½ head
	Carrots	6
	Brussels sprouts	6
	Broccoli	1 bunch
	Beets	2
	Bean sprouts	1½ cups
	Asparagus	8
	Spinach	2 cups
	Mushrooms	8
	Onions	1 medium
	Tomatoes	2
	Zucchini	2
	Lettuce	2 heads
	Parsley	1 bunch
	Radishes	10
Fruit	Apples	30
	Applesauce	15 cups
Fruit (cont.)	Bananas	15
	Cantaloupe	8 small
	Grapes	400
	Honeydew melon	4
	Oranges	30
	Orange juice	15 cups
	Pineapple	4
	Prunes	60
	Watermelon	25 cups
	Raisins	1 quart
Bread, starchy vegetables	Whole-wheat bread	45 slices
	Tortillas	20
	Bran flakes	10 cups
	Rice	10 cups
	Pasta	10 cups
	Popcorn	60 cups
	Flour	3 cups
	Waffles, 5"	20
	English muffins	10 whole
	Rye bread	13 slices
	Beans	10 cups
	Peas	10 cups
	Corn on the cob	20 small

Additional Food Required by a Woman (cont.)

Food Group	Item	Amount	Food Group	Item	Amount
	Potatoes	20 small	Fat (cont.)	Avocado	2
	Bagels	5 whole		Vegetable oil	½ cup
Meat and other protein foods	Beef, ground	2 pounds		Olives	100
	Chicken	2 pounds		Nuts	72
	Fish	3 pounds		Cream, heavy	1 cup
	Veal	1 pound		Cream cheese	1 cup
	Cheddar cheese	2 pounds		Salad dressing	1 cup
	Turkey	2 pounds		Mayonnaise	½ cup
	Eggs	27	Miscellaneous	Sugar, white	2 cups
	Cottage cheese	8 cups		Sugar, brown	2 cups
	Sardines	30		Sugar, syrup	2 cups
	Peanut butter	4 cups		Ice Cream	10 cups
	Beef roast	2 pounds		Dill pickles	40
Fat	Margarine	1 stick			

osteoporosis as they age. During the second trimester, when the infant's teeth start to develop, the presence of fluoride in prenatal supplements or in the diet increases the capacity of the child to withstand tooth decay when he or she is old enough to start eating candy. It also helps the tooth enamel withstand materials that erode the calcium, such as soft drinks and other acidic foods.

The expanding blood supply in the maternal tissue and the creation of the baby's blood volume make very great demands for iron. A woman's body typically contains 300 milligrams of stored iron. When she becomes pregnant instead of menstruating, she gains an additional 150 milligrams. But, even if this supply were to be transferred wholly to the needs of the fetus, it would be only half the amount needed. Therefore, the National Research Council recommends 30 to 60 milligrams of supplemental iron daily during pregnancy and for two to three months after delivery (see Chapter 8, Iron).

Protein intake must increase by 65 percent in order to satisfy the needs of the growing infant. The woman probably got along fine on 45 grams of high-quality protein before pregnancy, but she must now consume at least 75 or more grams.

Finally, constipation is a common problem during pregnancy, especially as the fetus gets bigger. The intestines become crowded by all the material that must now fit within the woman's abdomen, including the infant and the amniotic sac. Supplemental iron may add to constipation. It is best alleviated by two means: additional fiber and water, a combination that will maintain soft stools. Pregnant women have always been urged to eat plenty of roughage. A mild stimulant laxative can sometimes help as well, although laxatives should only be taken under the supervision of a physician.

All of these dietary additions are required to produce a normal, healthy infant. Mothers with poor diets run a great risk of complications, such as miscarriage, premature birth, and difficult deliveries. If the woman consumes a balanced diet and uses supplementation effectively, the nutritional challenges of pregnancy are a minor hurdle compared to the reward of a healthy child.

But how were all these special needs met in societies

where nutrition supplements were not available and supermarkets were not a few minutes away? As we have already learned in the case of the African termites, women through countless generations discovered ingenious ways to supplement their diets and passed these methods down.

In Chapter 8 I described European women pushing nails into apples, later removing the nails and eating the apple as a source of iron. Pregnancy, however, required a more powerful supplement. Women dissolved nails in vinegar and then used the vinegar as a sort of "soup stock." This was an effective mega-iron supplement.

In Chapter 9 I told about putting a "penny in the pickle jar." This was also used as a way of increasing the copper intake of mothers-to-be. From this may stem the folklore that pregnant women crave pickles.

One problem common to pregnant women in all cultures is the quest for extra calcium. This mineral is essential to the development of the child and to the health of the mother. In most societies there is some folklore associated with calcium intake and pregnant women, as in the saying, "Every child costs a tooth." If calcium intakes are inadequate during pregnancy, one of the first bones that gives up its calcium for the fetus is the alveolar bone of the lower jaw. This causes loosening of the teeth and invites periodontal disease, which often results in tooth loss: hence the saying.

The Asian cultures partially solved this problem by sweet-and-sour cooking. As we know, the "sour" in sweet-and-sour cooking, vinegar, leaches the calcium from the bones of whatever meat, poultry, or fish is used. Calcium was provided in other non-milk-drinking societies by simply grinding limestone and adding it to food.

Taboos in Pregnancy

Along with strange but effective dietary supplements, pregnancy has led to various taboos. These are red flags raised for serious purposes. In some societies women are forbidden to consume certain foods and beverages, especially stimulants. They are not allowed to consume alcoholic beverages or certain herbs which we know today contain strong laxatives or other chemicals that can cause a miscarriage. It's been felt from time to time that not allowing women to eat choice muscle meats was a plot on the part of male chauvinists to reserve the best cuts for themselves while leaving women to subsist as best they could on the organ meat. But, since organs such as liver and kidneys are such a rich source of the vitamins and minerals needed during pregnancy, this was actually a means of good nutrition.

Today we acknowledge the wisdom of many of the old taboos against ingesting certain substances during pregnancy. Extensive studies have shown that consumption of caffeine, alcohol, and tobacco can lead to serious problems. The results range from low birth weight to mental retardation and physical deformities. Cigarette smoking, for example, is known to lower birth weights (to 5½ pounds or less, whereas a normal baby weighs 6½ pounds or more). The difference may be only one pound but, as is often the case in nutrition, a small difference can be crucial. Birth weight is a key indicator of the baby's health. Low-birth-weight babies may be mentally retarded or short in stature for the rest of their lives.

In addition to smoking and malnutrition, inadequate weight gain during pregnancy could also cause a low birth weight. A woman may try to maintain a svelte figure even though she's pregnant, and rather than the prescribed 24 to 28 pounds she gains considerably less. Obviously, pregnancy is *not* the time to diet. A pregnant woman who goes on a fad diet—for example, a low-carbohydrate diet—runs the risk of increasing ketone bodies in the blood, which can cause mental retardation.

Alcohol is also toxic to the fetus and is eschewed by pregnant women in most societies. Some studies show that as little as one or two drinks a day impair mental development and cause specific physical deformities associated with fetal alcohol syndrome. However, even though this occurs in only one in 1,000 babies, it indicates that not all women can rely completely on instinct during pregnancy and must make a conscious effort to avoid alcohol.

Drugs during pregnancy should be regarded with great

caution. In the classic case, pregnant women who took a sedative called thalidomide gave birth to infants who were grotesquely deformed.

Many of these types of taboos were passed down but they also emerge as observations on the part of pregnant women. Many say, "The minute I became pregnant I knew there was something different because I just couldn't stand to drink any more coffee," or "I didn't want to drink any more alcohol," or "Somehow I just gave up smoking and I didn't need another cigarette." Are these sudden aversions instinctive? I think so. The body chemistry changes subtly and signals the brain that pregnancy has begun. Nature's need to protect its future takes over to preserve the health of the offspring.

Lactation

After the hurdle of the birth process has been cleared, the period of lactation is also nutritionally challenging. The infant's growth rate is astounding: weight doubles within the next six months and triples by the end of the first year (if the weight gain rate of the first six months continued, the child would weigh 7,000 pounds by its fifth birthday!). To support this rate of growth, high-quality nutrition is needed.

It's true that some nutrient requirements decline from their pregnancy level. For example, the mother's protein needs now drop 10 to 15 percent. After all, she is no longer growing almost 24 pounds of new tissue. But the infant's needs at this time are so great owing to intense growth that many requirements stay the same or even increase.

Caloric needs of the nursing mother outpace even those of pregnancy. The Food and Nutrition Board estimates she needs 500 calories' worth of additional food instead of 300 extra as in pregnancy. Even more may be needed later when the fat supplies of pregnancy are used up. Because water is needed to produce milk, ample fluid intake is important. Most mineral needs remain at the same high level; zinc and iodine even increase. While the great demand for folic acid drops, other vitamin needs increase slightly, especially the need for vitamins A and C. In fact, the infant needs 60 percent as much vitamin C as a full-grown man.

The vitamin content of the milk, especially the water-soluble vitamins, depends on the mother's vitamin intake. To an extent, as she eats so will her baby. But, as in pregnancy, nature favors the offspring, and if the demands for certain nutrients are not met by the mother's diet, they will come from her own tissues. This is particularly true for minerals.

It's important to recognize that the mother's calcium requirement remains as high during the period of nursing as it was during pregnancy. Some cultures had a taboo against a woman's going outside during the lactation period. This prolonged confinement prevented the nursing mother from getting out into the sun and, consequently, frustrated her body's ability to make vitamin D for the absorption of calcium. This meant that osteomalacia could develop—a vitamin D deficiency in adults that can lead to a softening of the bones. This taboo would have worked against reproductive success, not in its favor.

Mother's Milk

Human milk superbly meets all the infant's unique nutritional needs. If the mother's diet is anywhere near adequate, the infant's diet will be adequate because the composition of breast milk changes very little despite wide variations in the diet.

However, breast milk, beyond providing all the vitamins and minerals and macronutrients (protein, fat, and carbohydrates) needed for infant sustenance and growth, also meets some unusual nutritional needs. For example, during the last months of pregnancy vitamin E levels increase in the infant. As we explained in Chapter 4, vitamin E prevents the destruction of the red blood cells and the polyunsaturated fatty acids in the red blood cells. Human milk is high in the polyunsaturated fatty acid, linoleic acid, and once the infant is born and starts to nurse, vitamin E is there to protect the linoleic acid from oxidation and from the by-products of oxidation that can be harmful.

Human milk provides adequate, if not excellent, protection against disease. First, it contains certain protein materials that make nutrients available only to the infant. No microorganisms can feed on them. They literally preclude the ability of microorganisms to grow, so there is no danger of bacterial contamination as there is with other infant feeding sources. Secondly, the mother's milk contains a material called colostrum that passes antibodies from the mother into the baby's system during the first feedings only. It is a type of immunization system that will protect the infant from certain germs. Finally, certain components in the mother's milk stimulate the growth of beneficial microorganisms important to the production of intestinal flora in the growing infant. Human milk is unique in all these benefits for the human infant.

During the 1950s and 1960s scientifically developed infant formulas became enormously popular and doctors encouraged their use. Later research, however, revealed breast milk's inimitable superiority, and since the 1970s it has become the choice recommended by health professionals. One of breast milk's chief drawbacks is that nonnutritive substances consumed by the mother, such as caffeine, nicotine, artificial sweeteners, alcohol, aspirin, or some sedatives, can be passed into the milk. This can be avoided, though, by the conscientious mother.

Morning Sickness

Morning sickness often occurs early in pregnancy. It is likely to be similar to high-altitude sickness, a nausea brought on by a shortage of oxygen. In the case of morning sickness, it is caused by the rapidly developing tissues' outpacing the body's red-blood-cell supply (red blood cells transport oxygen throughout the body). It is very important during this period for the mother to have an adequate supply of all nutrients, especially iron, folic acid, and B_{12}, to enable her body to make the necessary amount of red blood cells.

In any case, morning sickness usually disappears after the first three months because by that time the mother's blood volume. has expanded to serve both her needs and the growing infant's; thus oxygen shortage no longer occurs.

The Rebound Scurvy Hypothesis

Recently a new phenomenon called rebound scurvy has been mentioned in some medical publications. It has been theorized that it could develop because of two different processes at work. Suppose a woman uses tremendous quantities of vitamin C (for example, 6 or 8 grams a day, which is 75 to 100 times the RDA for pregnant women) because she believes it is going to protect her and the fetus from colds. The vitamin C is quickly transferred across the placenta into the fetus's developing enzyme system. The infant becomes capable of metabolizing large quantities of vitamin C. After birth the infant consumes breast milk which, regardless of how much vitamin C the mother is ingesting, contains the normal amount of vitamin C required by the normal infant. But this infant's metabolic machinery has developed to metabolize large quantities of vitamin C very quickly. For all practical purposes, the infant quickly metabolizes itself into a situation of vitamin C deficiency even though it receives vitamin C in mother's milk. Some cases have been reported where infants affected in this way have developed some of the symptoms of scurvy.

Keep in mind that this subject needs additional studies before any conclusions can be drawn. But, until we know more about it, pregnant women should refrain from taking excessive levels of vitamin C.

Clearly, any pregnant or lactating woman should discuss her nutritional needs with her physician. If any medical practitioners are keenly aware of nutrition's impact on health, they are the obstetrician and pediatrician. They can offer the individual patient the best advice on nutritional supplementation for these crucial stages of infant development.

II

SODIUM AND POTASSIUM
The Critical Balance

When you're sick you think of chicken soup, not the canned or dry-mix kind, but the good, old-fashioned chicken soup that grandmother used to make. I'm talking about the soup nick-named "Jewish penicillin," although it probably originated in China. Chicken soup earned its reputation as a miracle drug by helping speed recovery from colds, flu, and the associated stomach upset, including vomiting or diarrhea, which is more than penicillin itself can do.

The soup does this in two ways. When made with chicken, fat, bones, and all the bone marrow, the soup releases certain aromatic compounds that speed the flow of mucus and help drain the mucous cavities. Second, the soup replaces vital electrolytes. During an extensive bout with cold and flu, or any illness involving diarrhea or vomiting, dehydration can occur, causing the loss of critical electrolytes such as potassium, sodium, and chloride. This prolongs the illness by hindering the efficient functioning of body systems and can even worsen the condition. Replacing the electrolytes helps speed recovery.

Can modern chicken soup from a can or package provide similar benefits? I don't think so, but I don't know for sure. The next time you get a cold or the flu or stomach upset and mild diarrhea, you may want to take chicken bones, some meat, fatty tissue such as the wings, and the flesh that clings to the bones, add some vegetables and a little salt and make a good, old-fashioned chicken soup. Spice it lightly and see if it doesn't seem to speed recovery.

Currents in the Body

This may sound strange to you, but your body contains electrically charged particles. That's why a doctor can take an electrocardiogram reading from your body, or why brushing your hair on a cold morning can make sparks fly, or why touching an exposed wire can be a shocking experience. You don't contain enough electricity to run an amplifier or even a lightbulb. We're not talking about household current here, but the relatively tiny potentials that send nerve impulses scurrying to their nerve receptors and back so your muscles react and thoughts turn into actions.

Certain mineral salts called electrolytes have the ability to dissolve in water and separate into their electrically charged particles, called ions. In this form they can conduct an electric current and thus make possible many nerve and muscle reactions, including the heartbeat. One ubiquitous electrolyte is sodium chloride, common table salt. Another is potassium chloride. Magnesium, which we covered in Chapter 7, is considered by some to be an electrolyte as well. Here we'll focus on sodium, which is supplied not only by salt but by milk, cheese, seafood, and other foods, and on potassium, especially high in such foods as dates, figs, peaches, blackstrap molasses, and raisins.

In addition to conducting electrical charges, the electrolytes provide another very important service for the body. Each of the body's trillions of cells is constantly bathed in fluids. There's two-way traffic through all the cell membranes. The blood and other fluids circulating outside the cells deliver nutrients, oxygen, and water to each and pick up the waste products each cell sends out. It is the electrolytes that regulate the movement of these important fluids in and out of the cells. If too much fluid left a cell, it would dehydrate; if too much rushed in, it would burst. The electrolytes maintain just the right level of fluid pressure.

In the fluids bathing the outside of the cell are sodium and chloride, while inside are potassium and a small amount of chloride. The balance between sodium and potassium is critically important to cell functions. These functions range from metabolizing certain materials to conducting nerve impulses that permit us to react to outside stimuli.

Too Much Salt of the Earth

A 150-pound person contains about eight ounces of potassium and three of sodium, a balance of over two to one in favor of potassium. Our ancestors almost certainly consumed a diet that had more potassium than sodium. Drs. S. Boyd Eaton and Melvin Konner state in a recent article that the overall ratio of potassium to sodium in the paleolithic diet was about 16 to 1. In this respect the caveman's diet was probably better than ours for, as we shall see, the modern American diet contains a ratio that is higher in sodium than potassium. Table salt is added extensively to many foods during processing and again by the consumer at meals. Not so for potassium.

Sodium has become a major problem in our society, not because it's scarce, but because we are drowning in a sea of salt. This wasn't always the case. In Roman times salt was so scarce that soldiers were paid with a salt ration. In fact, the word "salary" comes directly from the word "salt." Sayings such as "He is the salt of the earth" mean that a person is worthy and good. This indicates the high regard that people had in the past for salt. Salting food changes its taste, usually, it is felt, for the better. Most recipes instruct us to "salt to taste."

Nutritionists tell us the body needs an absolute minimum of 200 milligrams of sodium per day. As a safe and adequate range the government recommends 1,100 to 3,300 milligrams of sodium per day, and nearly half again as much potassium, 1,875 milligrams to 5,625 milligrams. Since sodium chloride (salt) is half chloride we can get our daily chloride requirement (1,700 to 5,100 milligrams) as well as that for sodium from our salt intake. The case for potassium is somewhat different, since we seldom, if ever, use potassium chloride in any pure form because of its metallic taste. We only get potassium from our food and gauge our intakes as so many milligrams per food item.

The average American diet may provide enough potassium, but vastly too much sodium. We are gorging on salt, actually debilitating our bodies with it. In place of the recommended 1,100 to 3,300 milligrams of sodium, we are ingesting 4,000 to 5,800 milligrams, corresponding to about 10 to 15 grams of salt. That's roughly two to six times too much.

This brings up the next question, "What does the body do with all this sodium?" To some extent the body can eliminate excess sodium. But, while it's still in the body, this enormous surplus of sodium creates an imbalance with the potassium available, even if the actual level of potassium is appropriate as measured against the *recommended* level of sodium. If we have too much sodium (from salt) in our blood, the body retains fluid to dilute the sodium. This is its way of trying to keep the concentration of sodium outside the cell in the correct proportion to potassium on the inside.

About 25 percent of adults have high blood pressure. It's caused by several factors, including heredity, but an imbalance of dietary sodium and potassium could be one of the culprits in sodium-sensitive people. People with high blood pressure are often treated with diuretics, which cause the body to eliminate fluid and with it excess sodium; unfortunately, some diuretics may also cause potassium losses.

The ideal diet would balance the intake of sodium with the intake of potassium. The problem is that we consume many highly processed foods that include tremendous amounts of sodium. A chicken breast might contain about 100 milligrams of sodium, which is less than 10 percent of the minimum daily requirement. But, if we purchase the same piece of chicken at a fast-food outlet, where it has been seasoned and fried in grease, we find that it now contains about 900 milligrams of sodium. In other words, the sodium content has increased by a factor of nine, with no increase in potassium.

And so it is with many of our foods. Become a label reader, remembering that ingredients on processed foods are listed in descending order of their amount. For example, on the label of breakfast cereals or other processed foods, salt may appear as one of the first three or four ingredients. In canned foods, water or the vegetable may be the first ingredient and various forms of sugar often come next. If salt follows it, think twice.

Commonly used dried soup mixes in the supermarket contain, on a dry-weight basis, approximately 10 percent salt. If the package contents weigh 1 ounce (approximately 30 grams) and consist of 10 percent salt, that's approximately 3 grams of salt. If the package makes about 4 servings, each bowl would contain about 1.75 grams of salt. That's about 300 milligrams of sodium, whereas the amount of potassium in the same food would be less than 100 milligrams. To add insult to injury, many people make the soup at twice the recommended concentration. In this case, a single bowl would contain over half of the daily allotment of sodium.

In contrast, old-fashioned chicken soup contained more potassium than sodium. This is true of most natural vegetables, fruits, even meats—they provide more potassium than sodium. In fact, if traditional chicken soup were being newly developed today it might be marketed as an "electrolyte supplement."

Where Has All the Potassium Gone?

Just about every food on the earth was relatively moderate in sodium until civilization put its stamp on it through food processing. For example:

- Crab contains 300 milligrams of potassium and 200 milligrams of sodium per serving, obviously an excellent ratio. However, canned crab contains only 100 milligrams of potassium and 1,000 milligrams of sodium.
- A frankfurter contains 100 milligrams of potassium, which is not bad, but it's also loaded with 550 milligrams of sodium. That's excessive!
- Most cheeses that are "processed" rather than fermented contain more sodium than potassium. American cheese, a completely processed cheese, contains 300 milligrams of sodium and only 25 milligrams of potassium.
- Bakery products normally contain more sodium than they do potassium, in part because baking soda and baking powder are

both high in sodium, in part because commercially-baked goods usually contain salt.

• In the popular breakfast cereals, the ratio is again in favor of sodium.

Use some common sense. Nature seems to provide the right balance of sodium and potassium. It's the processed-food industry that gets this all out of balance. So when in doubt resort to natural foods—fresh foods, vegetables, fruits, grains. In the main, these foods contain large amounts of potassium, whereas they contain relatively minor amounts of sodium. Apples, bananas, cantaloupes, and grapes all are potassium-rich. Vegetables are also great sources. Celery contains 50 milligrams of sodium per serving, which is relatively minor, and 130 milligrams of potassium. Fresh tomato juice has a very good sodium/potassium ratio, as does canned salt-free tomato juice. However, when tomato juice is processed with salt, the amount of sodium per 100 grams rises from only 3 milligrams to around 200! Similarly, cucumbers contain only 6 milligrams of sodium per 100 grams and 155 milligrams of potassium. Once those cucumbers are processed into dill pickles, the sodium content shoots up to 1,428 milligrams.

Here are some more examples of healthy sodium/potassium ratios you'll find in natural foods:

Food (100 gm)	Sodium (mg)	Potassium (mg)
Apple	1	110
Banana	1	370
Broccoli, cooked	10	267
Carrot, raw	47	341
Date, dry	1	648
Orange	1	272
Spinach, cooked, no salt	50	324
Tomato, raw	3	244

From USDA 1963.

The increased consumption of processed foods has contributed to the declining potassium content in our diet. Equally important, it has altered the ratio of sodium to potassium in the unfavorable direction of increased sodium. Sodium is an integral part of food processing; potassium is not. In addition to salt, many food additives in processed foods contain sodium. Sodium nitrite, found often in luncheon meats and bacon, is one; sodium benzoate, a common soft-drink ingredient, is another. Fresh foods are where we get our potassium. If a person does not consume adequate daily servings of fresh foods, especially vegetables, he or she won't get sufficient potassium.

Remember that if one serving of a food contains about 200 to 300 milligrams of potassium you have to have four to five or more servings to meet your daily needs. In contrast you can get more than enough sodium, usually, in just one, or at most two, servings of a processed food.

Theories on Hypertension

This is one of the major problems of civilization. If we examine nonindustrialized primitive societies with diets abundant in fresh foods, high blood pressure generally is almost nonexistent. If these same people move into a modern-day society, their blood pressure usually creeps up.

For example, in a classic study scientists noted that natives in small villages in New Guinea had virtually no hypertension. The old men had the same blood-pressure levels as young men. Yet natives from these villages nearly always developed hypertension when they moved to modern coastal cities. Similarly, when East African Samburu herdsmen were at home tending their flocks and eating 50 milligrams of sodium daily, they had very little hypertension. However, when they were drafted into the army of Kenya and ate army rations, their blood pressure became progressively elevated.

High blood pressure is one of the major risk factors in heart disease and stroke. It's also involved in kidney failure, although it's not clear which comes first, the kidney failure or the high blood pressure.

The risk factors possibly leading to high blood pressure are several.

1. There is a hereditary component. Regardless of their diet some people inherit high blood pressure. In this case, there doesn't seem to be much to do except use various medications and follow a restricted sodium diet.
2. A major risk factor for high blood pressure is excess weight. When a person gains weight his or her blood pressure may become elevated. In many cases, simply reducing weight down to normal is sufficient to eliminate the high blood pressure.
3. Excess sodium is the other risk factor. As dietary sodium increases so does blood pressure in susceptible people. Some people with high blood pressure can consume sodium without adverse effects, but most cannot—to them it's like poison.
4. Excessive alcohol consumption also elevates blood pressure in susceptible individuals.

Today there is some new evidence that reduced intakes of calcium and potassium as well as excess sodium intake seem to play a role in the development of high blood pressure in susceptible individuals (see p. 91). Much more research is needed on the calcium hypothesis, so don't let it sidetrack you from moderating your sodium intake.

Blood Pressure Measurements and What They Mean

When your blood pressure is measured you get two numbers, "systolic over diastolic." The systolic refers to the pressure when your heart is actually pumping and diastolic is the pressure when your heart rests between beats. If your systolic blood pressure is over 160 or your diastolic blood pressure is over 90, when you are resting, you should see your physician. About 25 percent of U.S. adults have high blood pressure. As Americans get past the age of sixty-five, three out of four have high blood pressure.

When children have high blood pressure it could be an inherited problem. Most physicians or medical experts today agree that children of parents who have high blood pressure should be raised on a diet that's relatively low in salt. The same, of course, can be said about other dietary factors relevant in cases of diabetes, obesity, and some other diseases.

Blood pressure is a way of measuring how hard your heart has to pump to get all your blood through the body so it can perform its functions. If you put on a pound of extra weight, there's about a mile of capillaries and blood vessels that have to be developed. It's easy to see that the heart is going to have to pump harder to get that blood through those extra passageways. Obesity's effect on blood pressure is easily understood. However, the connection with sodium is not quite as obvious. There seem to be a couple of possible explanations, each of which we will consider in turn.

First, retention of fluid will cause high blood pressure in its own right. People who consume large amounts of salt retain more fluid and this could elevate their blood pressure. By retaining fluid, the body dilutes the sodium concentration. When people who have developed this condition reduce their salt intake substantially, they often lose some weight because, as the sodium content of their body drops, so does the fluid content. As long as they stay on a reduced sodium diet they'll help to keep that weight off.

Heredity is always a major factor in high blood pressure. Some people inherit the tendency, which may be triggered by a dietary imbalance of sodium and potassium. But, once the high blood pressure has developed, a low-sodium diet will not always solve the problem. Even so, a low-sodium diet may help to reduce the amount of medication required.

One of the major treatments for high blood pressure is a diuretic, a medication to help eliminate body fluids. By eliminating body fluids, diuretics also help eliminate excess amounts of sodium contained in the fluids. The problem with diuretics is that some of them also may cause the excretion of potassium. Make sure the diet is loaded with fresh fruits and vegetables high in potassium and, if necessary, discuss the use of a potassium supplement with a physician.

What Can We Do Ourselves?

Although science is still studying high blood pressure, it's important that we take steps ourselves to use what we know to prevent or control this life-threatening disease. As we go into the last fifteen years of this twentieth century we know that there are certain steps that are fundamental in reducing blood pressure: reduce weight to normal; reduce sodium intake to about 2 grams per day (that's 5 grams of salt); maintain a diet that supplies more potassium than sodium as well as adequate and balanced amounts of all the other minerals, such as calcium; and consume alcohol in moderation.

If blood pressure remains high the physician can control it with medication, which may be kept to a minimum with proper diet. This doesn't imply that the person with very high blood pressure shouldn't be put on medication immediately, only that most of us should strive to control our weight and diet to see if we can eliminate high blood pressure without the use of diuretics.

Water, Water Everywhere

The most critically important nutrient required by most living creatures on this earth is oxygen; the second most important nutrient is water. The actual water requirement of a body depends on size and lifestyle. For example, a person working in an oil rig in the desert will require more water than a person sitting at a desk in a New York City office. And a 250-pound person will require more water than a 150-pound person doing the same thing.

We can go without many nutrients for long periods of time, some for months and some for a year, but without water for only a very short period of time. The adult body is approximately 60 percent water. We start our life being about 80 percent water, so that on a body-weight basis the infant requires more water than the adult. Depending on what the individual does, an adult requires approximately four to eight glasses of water per day (it can be even higher than that if one is an athlete working under conditions of low humidity, high heat, and tremendous energy output). We may go for weeks without ever drinking a glass of plain water, but we consume water in many different ways, in coffee, tea, beverages, and in our foods. Most fruits and vegetables are 85 to 95 percent water. Even bread is 30 to 35 percent water.

The perils of dehydration are numerous but the most common is that the blood becomes more viscous, the flow through the arteries is more difficult, and blood pressure goes up.

Under extreme dehydration potassium starts to leave the cells, and we know from this chapter that potassium is absolutely necessary *inside* the body cells—all of them, from brain cells to the cells of the big toe. Extreme potassium deficiency can develop from excessive use of certain diuretics without a counterbalancing intake of potassium. This may also happen when people go on a low-calorie diet that is inadequate in potassium. Cells simply cannot function properly. In the case of a heart cell it means that the heart can't beat properly owing to a potassium deficiency within the heart cells themselves or within the nerve cells that send the signals that tell the heart to beat; in the case of a nerve cell the nerve doesn't function properly. The net result can be death. So potassium deficiency can be extremely dangerous. The same would be true of sodium deficiency, but this almost never occurs. When a baby's diet changes to family foods in our society, its salt intake triples or quadruples.

You Are the Lifeguard

We may be drowning in a sea of salt, but we don't have to. Each of us is, in a sense, a lifeguard. You have control over what you eat. Think about it. The life you save may be your own.

In nature most foods are born low-sodium foods and they are well balanced in sodium and potassium. Consequently, if you eat lots of fresh fruits, vegetables, meats, and poultry you really don't have to worry. Go sparingly on gravy and salty condiments such as soy sauce and MSG. Experiment with lemon juice and herbs instead.

If you eat processed foods, remember any processed high-protein products, such as frankfurters, sausage, salami, luncheon meats, or fried chicken from a fast-food carryout are very high in sodium. If you use canned food, select those that are specifically labeled as low sodium, such as low-sodium soup, low-sodium vegetables, or low-sodium tuna, and rinse the contents with water. Recognize that we can't wholly avoid the use of processed foods, since one of the things that characterizes our society is the tendency toward "convenience."

Actually, salt was one of the earliest preservatives; it was originally added to canned foods to prevent the growth of bacteria. Similarly, people salted meat to prevent the growth of microorganisms. In dry foods salt also reduces what food technologists call "water activity," which also prevents bacterial growth. Nowadays, because of refrigeration we don't require all that salt, but it's still used.

Most of us tend to think that normal or average means okay. Yet we know that high blood pressure is not healthy. So, when three out of four people over sixty-five in our country have high blood pressure we must ask ourselves, how can we avoid being "normal"? If three out of four people were insane, would we lock up the sane people and say that insanity is okay because it's normal?

In the case of blood pressure, being normal can kill you. As a society we are doing something wrong. Too many of us are overweight, and too many of us still eat too many high-sodium processed foods and too little fresh food. These are factors we can change. Each of us should take personal action no matter what our age to make sure that being a normal American means being a healthy American.

12

FISH OILS, FATS, AND GARLIC
The Cholesterol Problem

Ever since modern health science discovered the connection between fat and heart attack, the Greenland Eskimos have been a mystery. Here is a group of people that defy the laws of healthy eating by consuming a very high-fat diet. Yet they have an astonishingly low rate of heart disease and stroke.

To solve the mystery, several teams of epidemiologists conducted extensive research studies during the 1970s and early 1980s. They came up with a revolutionary finding. Fat can be good for the heart. It depends on what kind of fat.

The Eskimos get much of their oil from salmon, mackerel, and cod, which live in cold water. The oil in these fish contains a special fatty acid that may be the clue to the Eskimos' healthy hearts. It's called eicosapentaenoic acid—EPA for short. We'll soon discuss EPA and its implications for health. Suffice it to say for now that the types of fats prominent in our Western diet don't contain a drop of this oily substance. Given our heart-attack rate, maybe we should give it some thought.

Everyone no doubt has heard the old folk saying "Fish is brain food." People still cite it to encourage children to eat fish. No one has ever fully understood what this aphorism means. One school of thought suggests that fish is considered brain food because of the similarity in color and texture between fish meat and the human brain. I don't think so. I think the ancients understood something about fish oil that science has just rediscovered.

When the blood circulating throughout the body becomes too thick with accumulated fats, certain particles in blood called platelets become sticky and can clump together inside the blood vessel. This may develop into a devastating blood clot that can result in a stroke or heart attack. If stroke victims survive, many of their brain functions are usually gone for good. They may be paralyzed, unable to walk, talk, or even feed themselves.

Over generations, people probably observed that those who frequently ate fish not only lived longer but went to their graves with their brains intact, avoiding not only strokes but senility. Hence, the saying.

Now that some of these anecdotal observations are beginning to attract scientific support, it may be possible to consider fish oils as well as certain other oils as kinds of nutrients. Most of these oils are not essential to life in the same way as, say, vitamin C. But they do help the body deal with the unhealthy shift to fat in our diet. Thus, these oils could be beneficial to the health of major segments of the population.

In order to understand EPA and other fish oils and how our lifestyles may have created a role for them, let's take a closer look at the other fats and oils familiar to all of us.

Why You Need Fat

Chances are you've probably never had a meal that didn't contain some fat. Whether it's beef fat dripping from a hamburger, butter or margarine spread on a roll, olive or corn oil dressing a salad, or cream making dessert moist, fats show up at every meal.

Fat is simple to detect. You can spot it by the translucent shiny spot it leaves on paper (always a telltale sign on bags containing greasy doughnuts or fast foods). Fat is greasy to the touch and cannot be dissolved in water. Among nutritionists and other scientists, fats are also called lipids, and the clinical name for too much fat in the blood is hyperlipidemia. All fats are lipids, but not all lipids are fats. For example, lecithin is a lipid but it is not a fat. The fat-soluble vitamins, A, D, E, and K, also belong to the lipid family.

We eat about a quarter pound of fat each day. Fat accounts for over 40 percent of the food energy we consume, too much by most health professionals' standards. The recommended level is 30 percent.

Fat has become a dirty word, but this dietary component fulfills specific functions in the body that no other nutrient can. Because it does not mix easily with water, the fatty tissues of the body can absorb and store substances such as the fat-soluble vitamins. Fat acts as a concentrated energy reserve, providing more calories per gram than any other nutrient. It offers protection and, to some degree, thermal insulation for delicate inner organs. In these ways and others, fat is helpful to us.

Fatty acids are vital to the life of all of our cells. Along with certain lipids they play extremely important roles in an impressive list of body functions. These include enzyme reactions, synthesis and regulation of hormones, maintenance of blood vessels, energy metabolism, digestion, formation of cell membranes and tissues, transmission of nerve impulses, and memory.

All fats contain fatty acids but the type depends upon the source of fat. For example, the Eskimos' EPA is a fatty acid found in the fat of cold-water fish. You wouldn't find it in pork fat or chicken fat. Only one fatty acid is now thought to be essential —needed for life but unable to be synthesized by the body. It's called linoleic acid. If the body has enough, it can make all the *other* fatty acids needed for critical body functions.

Although there is no RDA for fatty acids, the U.S. Food and Nutrition Board states that our linoleic-acid intake needs to be 2 percent of total energy consumed. This equals about a tablespoon of vegetable oil. Unfortunately, most of us consume far more fat than we need, and of the wrong kind at that.

Good Fats, Bad Fats

Fat comes in two basic kinds. Depending on how many hydrogen atoms their chemical structures contain, fats are classified as "saturated" or "unsaturated." Although seemingly a minor molecular difference, hydrogen in fat makes all the difference in the world to human health.

All that a nonscientist really needs to know is that saturated fats are those found in animal products such as hamburger, bacon, cheese, ice cream, and butter. Unsaturated fats are generally found in plants, which are converted, for example, into vegetable oil, margarine, and peanut butter (coconut provides a perplexing exception to the rule; it is a plant yet its fat is highly saturated). Some plant fats (mostly seed oils) are extremely high in polyunsaturated fats, while olive oil contains a fairly large amount of monounsaturated fats together with some polyunsaturated. Most oils are unsaturated fats.

Saturated fats tend to be solid at room temperature while unsaturated fats are liquid and clear. Compare the hard white fat around the edge of a cut of meat or the fat marbled through it to a bottle of clear, golden corn oil.

Saturated fats can literally clog up the works—namely the arteries—whereas polyunsaturated and monounsaturated oils circulate through the body with ease and don't appear to cause unhealthy fat buildup in the blood.

But unsaturated oils can be transformed into solid saturated fats by a process known as "hydrogenation." Vegetable shortening and margarine are two well-known partially hydrogenated products. Even though they do not contain cholesterol, they may be less healthful than the same oils in their natural liquid form. But consuming small amounts of saturated fats is not harmful.

Hidden Fats

Whether saturated or unsaturated, 40 percent of the fat in the American diet comes from visible sources such as butter, margarine, salad dressing, and mayonnaise. But the remaining 60 percent lurks as "hidden" fat in meat, dairy products, sauces, convenience foods, and pastries. A pie crust, for example, gets its prized flaky texture and fine flavor from fat. A low-fat food such as potatoes can be converted into the high-fat food called potato chips. Another sad example is shrimp. Fresh shrimp contain about 10 percent fat, but, breaded and fried, their fat content jumps to 50 percent.

Food manufacturers routinely add fat to processed foods

to make them more tasty. Snack crackers are close to 40 percent fat, and powdered coffee whiteners or nondairy creamers weigh in at about 50 percent fat. Fat wouldn't be added to our foods if it didn't sell, but perhaps it will sell less as consumers learn more about nutrition.

Why do we like fat so much? Part of it is taste. As it has developed the sweet tooth, our society has cultivated a craving for the pleasurable sensation, the smooth creaminess, that fat provides. That's why we'll take a low-fat food like fish and deep-fat fry it, then smother it with gooey tartar sauce. We like to spread thick dressings on our salads and sour cream on our potatoes. Most people prefer whole milk to lowfat milk.

Another reason we like fat is that it slows down the emptying time of the stomach. That's why fatty meals give you that nice "full" feeling (although too much fat can cause discomfort). In contrast Chinese food contains relatively little fat, just bits of meat instead of large hunks, and no buttery sauces. That's one of the reasons why you can eat in a Chinese restaurant and feel hungry an hour later. A high-carbohydrate meal is easily cleared through the digestive system, and this is good for your health.

The amount of fat in a person's diet seems to depend on affluence. It's a matter of whether land and other resources can be spared to raise animals, as in the U.S., or whether all available land needs to be used for grain cultivation for food, such as rice in Asia.

In poor Asian nations, the fat content of the diet can be as low as 10 percent. In the U.S., the fat content of our meals has increased steadily since the 1920s, and so has our heart-attack rate. Currently in such nations as the Netherlands, Denmark, New Zealand, Canada, and the U.S., where dairy products, meats, and vegetable oils are available at prices most people can afford, fats account for 40 to 45 percent of the diet. Thus, it's the affluent who suffer most from heart disease and diseases associated with overweight, such as diabetes, and hypertension.

Atherosclerosis

In Western countries cardiovascular disease, which includes heart attack and stroke, has reached epidemic proportions. In the United States, despite a modest decrease in recent years, cardiovascular disease is still the leading cause of death, with a mortality rate twice that of cancer, the second-largest cause of death (Chapter 13).

One of the underlying causes of cardiovascular disease is the condition called atherosclerosis, a narrowing of the arteries due to a buildup of cholesterol and fat along the artery walls. A blood clot can form in one of these narrow spaces, closing up the artery and cutting off the flow of blood to the tissue it serves. If the tissue happens to be in the brain or heart, a stroke or heart attack occurs. Sometimes, a blood clot from another part of the body can become dislodged, move through the circulatory system, and reach the heart or brain with the same result.

Unlike an infectious disease such as influenza or smallpox, atherosclerosis does not strike overnight. It takes years for a fatal amount of fat to build up. American men tend to start dying of heart attacks in their mid-forties, a period when most men are in their prime as husbands, fathers, and workers. Biology seems to protect women until menopause, but in their fifties their heart-disease rate catches up with that of men.

Atherosclerosis has been linked to many factors, including obesity, smoking, high blood pressure, and a family history of heart disease or stroke. Some people think a sense of time urgency, known as "Type A behavior," is involved. Certainly, it's also linked to high levels of fat and cholesterol in the blood. However, as we saw in the case of the Greenland Eskimos, it's not only fat intake per se that does the damage, but a particular type of fat consumed. Higher intakes of saturated fatty acids as compared to polyunsaturated fatty acids, and higher cholesterol intake tend to raise the risk of heart disease.

As with fatty acids, so with cholesterol—there are many types, with very different consequences for health. Recently the scientific spotlight has focused on the risk associated with the type of cholesterol called LDL, short for "low density lipoproteins." It is this type of cholesterol that is deposited in the arteries. Elevated levels of LDL cholesterol usually mean there's a higher risk of heart disease.

The "good" kind of cholesterol seems to be HDL, short for "high density lipoprotein." HDL cholesterol reduces the risk of heart disease. Thus, it is desirable to have a higher level of HDL in the blood than of LDL. This is not as confusing as it seems. Generally speaking, the same factors we associate with reducing the risk of heart disease, higher intakes of polyunsaturated fatty acids, lower intakes of saturated fats, exercise, moderating alcohol intake, and correcting obesity, all seem to increase the ratio of HDL to LDL cholesterol in the blood.

Lowering high blood pressure is important, too, in reducing the risk of heart disease and stroke. Blood coursing through the arteries at high pressure can cause an injury to one of the blood vessels. Plaque can accumulate at the site of the injury just the way a scab forms on a cut on the outside of your body. The difference is that when a scab's work is done it can simply fall off the skin, but inside a blood vessel plaque has nowhere to go.

When genetic factors are at work, altering diet may not always be effective. But, while genetic factors are beyond our control, we *can* control what we eat. Taking charge of your health to the best of your abilities is important to the well-being of every individual.

How easily one's blood tends to form clots is also thought to be an important factor in heart disease and stroke. Just in the last decade, scientists have discovered dietary factors that may reduce clotting. These, like the EPA in the fish Eskimos eat, tend to be polyunsaturated fatty acids.

We will now take an in-depth look at the fatty acids that seem to be generating the most excitement because of their apparent ability to lower cholesterol, reduce clotting, or both.

EPA

Cold-water fish, like all other creatures, need fat and fatty acids. But in order to be useful the fats must stay liquid despite the freezing temperatures of the world's northern ocean currents. Polyunsaturated fats like EPA do the trick for salmon, mackerel, anchovies, sardines, and others.

Fish don't actually make EPA. It occurs in simple ocean organisms, such as plankton, that fish eat.

As we noted earlier, a diet rich in this marine fatty acid is one of the reasons, some researchers believe, Greenland Eskimos have such a low rate of heart disease and stroke. Further studies revealed that the Eskimos indeed have very low levels of unhealthy fats in their blood and high levels of good HDL cholesterol. It was further found that EPA slows down blood platelets' function in clot formation.

Danish scientists have compared the bleeding times of Greenland Eskimos and Danes, who consume a diet high in saturated fats. Sure enough, the diet containing the highly polyunsaturated fatty acid EPA gave the Eskimos a longer bleeding time or, you might say, "thinner" blood. Blood slower to clot on the outside is a good indicator of blood less likely to form potentially fatal clots on the inside.

And you don't have to be an Eskimo to reap benefits from EPA. Studies on volunteers in Sweden and in Oregon both came up with decreased blood clotting and longer bleeding times in those consuming fish rich in EPA. In the latter study, after ten days on a salmon diet, healthy volunteers showed a 15 percent decrease in LDL cholesterol and a 45 percent decrease in other fats in the blood. The decrease for people who started the study with abnormally high cholesterol and fat levels was even more dramatic. Similarly, blood viscosity was found to be much lower among Japanese living in coastal fishing villages with intakes of fish high in EPA than among inland Japanese farming villagers.

EPA as part of a total dietary plan designed to modify fat

and cholesterol intake may reduce blood cholesterol levels and help increase the ratio of HDL to LDL.

Despite our mothers' urging that fish is "brain food," hardly anyone eats oily blue-skinned fish once a week, let alone once a day. EPA supplementation may be appropriate.

DHA

DHA is an abbreviation for docosahexaenoic acid, a fatty acid found in salted and fresh cold-water fish in association with EPA. It is also found in the human brain. Unfortunately, the workings of that delicate white and gray matter we call the brain is an area where twentieth-century scientific knowledge is still woefully incomplete. DHA can be acquired directly from the diet or metabolized from the fatty acid linoleic acid. Human milk is rich in DHA because the infant brain must acquire its mass of DHA after birth. Further details about DHA remain to be discovered.

Linoleic Acid

What EPA is to plant life in the ocean, linoleic acid is to land plants. Plants contain this polyunsaturated fatty acid and lucky thing for us that they do. Linoleic acid is the one fatty acid now known to be essential for human life. One way that we know it's essential is that human breast milk contains it in generous amounts, in the highest concentration among all mammals, in fact. You never outgrow your need for linoleic acid. A complete lack of linoleic acid in the diet during any stage of life can produce deficiency symptoms, another classic sign of essentiality.

Vegetable oils and wheat-germ oils are very rich in linoleic acid. Margarine, nuts, poultry, and fish are also good sources. Another good source of linoleic acid is the lipid called lecithin. Lecithin is unusual because it contains fatty acids and a nonfat component, phosphorus. It is a phospholipid and not a fat. Lecithin is found in egg yolk and organ meats, two very high-cholesterol sources. Although whole grains contain some lecithin, soybean lecithin is the richest cholesterol-free source. Lecithin extracted from soybean oil can provide a low-calorie, cholesterol-free source of linoleic acid.

Increasing linoleic acid in the diet and decreasing saturated fats has been shown to significantly lower cholesterol levels, shift LDL to HDL cholesterol, and optimize blood viscosity.

Garlic Oil

When a plague outbreak occurred in eighteenth-century London, French and English priests alike were busy tending the sick and dying. But somehow only the English priests caught the disease. Apparently the French priests' health was safeguarded by their routine consumption of garlic.

Since the beginning of recorded history—in Sanskrit documents in India, scrolls in China, and Egyptian papyruses—garlic has been praised as both a culinary herb and therapeutic agent.

Across the centuries, noteworthy healers have employed garlic. The Greek physician Galen acclaimed the "stinking rose" as the commonfolk's "heal-all." Hippocrates prescribed it for everything from constipation to uterine tumors. And Pliny, the Roman naturalist, recommended garlic as treatment for more than sixty disorders.

But although garlic's culinary worth has never been questioned, claims about its healing powers are certainly controversial. Herbalists have always stood by garlic, but modern scientists once looked askance at what they considered to be quaint folklore. Today, however, scientific evidence is beginning to indicate that garlic may be good for warding off more than vampires. In addition to being effective for some bacterial and fungus infections, garlic may play a role in warding off heart disease.

Studies in India show that members of a sect who eat lots of garlic and onions have significantly lower levels of blood cholesterol and other fats than those whose diets are low in these plants. Further research indicates that garlic can reduce cholesterol levels by as much as 17 percent.

Garlic research in the U.S. began in 1944 with the chemical isolation of an oil from crushed garlic. This oil contains active ingredients such as allicin, short for allyl sulphide. Allicin gives garlic not only its odor but probably also its antibacterial attributes.

Garlic oil's use as an antibiotic dates back for centuries. Garlic has also been used as a preservative for meats and other foods, because it prevents the growth of bacteria and mold. As recently as World War I garlic juice was used to sterilize wounds and prevent infection.

Garlic's possible anticholesterol role was first investigated by a scientist at Philadelphia's Wistar Institute, who became intrigued by his aged but youthful landlady's claim that the garlic she ate daily was responsible for her good health. His studies found that in addition to lowering cholesterol, garlic can slow the development of atherosclerotic plaque and inhibit blood clots.

Similar findings have emerged from other universities and the USDA's Human Nutrition Center. Researchers who expected to find that allicin (the antibacterial factor) was also the anticlotting factor were surprised to find the latter role filled by another chemical, called adenosine.

Unfortunately, it seems the beneficial components of garlic are also the odorous parts. Although "odorless" garlic pills are available, their therapeutic potency is untested. Chemists who have analyzed some of these pills claim they are frauds, containing only a drop of garlic oil mixed with plain vegetable oil. In addition, the processing methods used to make other garlic products, such as powders, pills, and extracts, sometimes seem to destroy the active ingredients. Also, at this point the amount required for beneficial effects in humans seems very high. Reportedly one would have to consume half a bulb daily, an intake that would require tolerance from co-workers and friends.

University scientists are presently at work developing a pharmacologically active garlic derivative. More studies are underway to explain garlic's effect on blood.

Researchers in the U.S. are obviously far from ready to recommend a bulb a day to keep the doctor away, but it couldn't hurt. Garlic can provide a low-calorie, low-sodium way to enhance food flavor and possibly do much more.

The Evening-Primrose-Oil Controversy

The evening primrose is a large, delicate wildflower native to North America and is not a true primrose. The blooms usually last only one evening, at which time they are pollinated by flying insects. The power of evening primrose lies in its tiny seeds, which hold an oil rich in gamma-linoleic acid (GLA). GLA exists in humans as an intermediary fatty acid. It is metabolized from the essential fatty acid linoleic acid, in order to produce the biologically active prostaglandins. These are hormonelike substances that participate in such diverse reactions as gastric secretions, blood-pressure regulation, hormone release, and smooth-muscle contractions, including those of the uterus.

Although evening-primrose oil may have some value, the studies are still too few and too preliminary to make any firm conclusions.

Research by Dr. D. F. Horrobin has found that some women who suffer from the discomfort of premenstrual syndrome have lower than normal levels of GLA. He further showed that GLA may reduce irritability and pain in these women.

Various factors, it appears, may block the body's ability to metabolize linoleic acid into GLA. These include alcohol consumption, high cholesterol intake, diabetes mellitus, aging, lack of zinc, viral infections, and poor dietary sources of linoleic acid, such as highly processed vegetable oils. Theoretically, GLA can fit right into the chain of reactions that form prostaglandins, thus filling a metabolic gap for some people who may be unable to metabolize linoleic acid to GLA or who have low dietary intakes of linoleic acid.

There is some limited evidence produced by Dr. J. Chaintreul that GLA can to some extent reduce blood cholesterol levels. But it is unclear at this time whether this is true only for people who may have had a predisposition to high cholesterol because of chronic diseases.

Hopefully, more studies will be forthcoming in the near

future. Until then evening-primrose oil and its possible benefits must remain a subject of controversy.

Polyunsaturated-Fat Deficiencies

Gone are the days when clearcut deficiency symptoms made it easy to define nutrients. Today we must contend with a cluster of subtle, complicated symptoms, such as internal blood clots, narrowed arteries, and elevated fats and cholesterol in the blood. If that weren't bad enough, we now have to distinguish between more than one type of cholesterol.

Maybe our concept of what defines a nutrient needs to change. Maybe under special circumstances certain fatty acids may be critical for some people, say those with elevated blood cholesterol or problems such as premenstrual syndrome. Perhaps our highly saturated Western diets have created a situation where adding these polyunsaturated fatty acids to our diet is important for longevity and health.

At present we can only speculate about this. Unlike other deficiencies, decades may pass before a deficiency of polyunsaturated fatty acids takes its toll on a person's health, thus making clinical studies out of the question. Research will continue, but in the interim perhaps we should all try to substitute some polyunsaturated fatty acids for part of the saturated fatty acids in the diet. Someday we may be very glad that we did.

13

CANCER

Dietary Factors

Cancer is one of the major scourges of our civilization. As many diseases caused by infective agents have become curable, cancer has increased in relative importance. This would have happened even if our exposure to cancer-causing substances had remained constant. However, this exposure has increased. Whether we consider radiation, pesticides, certain additives or preservatives, the thousands of other chemicals synthesized by modern industry, or the practice of inhaling smoke from burning tobacco, we are surrounded by potential carcinogens. As a result, the incidence of certain types of cancer has increased by leaps and bounds during the twentieth century.

Cancer has been with us for a long time indeed, probably as long as humanity. We know that animals and fish also get cancer, so it is probably one of the forms of pestilence associated with living things since the dawn of time. For example, bodies buried five hundred or more years ago in Greenland or over two thousand years in other parts of the world have shown evidence of malignant tumors. Our forefathers suffered from what they called "the wasting disease." Think of people wasting away: what comes to mind is starvation. When people die of cancer they usually suffer from severe starvation, since the cancer takes all the nourishment. Consequently they appear to "waste away." Before our eyes a young person can become so weakened by cancer that he is unable even to lift his head from the pillow of his deathbed.

In our time, some components of the typical diet appear

to promote cancer. By removing those things from the diet, each of us may reduce the risk of cancer. In the case of other dietary components, a deficiency may increase the risk of cancer, so ingesting adequate amounts is important.

The causes of cancer are unbelievably complex, involving not only diet but also lifestyle, working conditions, heredity, and other factors. In the U.S. some 870,000 people will have developed some type of cancer in 1984. It is second only to heart disease in fatalities of its victims. Although heart disease is feared by everyone, cancer is the most dreaded of all diseases. Cancer strikes more frequently as people grow older, but it affects people of all ages; it kills more children than any other disease. Statistics show that about 30 percent of all people in the United States will get cancer before they die. That's about 67,000,000 Americans. To look at it another way, cancer will ultimately strike someone in three out of four families living in the United States today.

Of all the types of cancer, lung cancer is probably the most widely known, but digestive-system-related cancers strike more people. In 1984, cancer of the colon, rectum, and other digestive organs accounted for more cases than lung cancer. In addition, breast cancer (accounting for 116,000 cases), prostate cancer, and cancer of the uterus may have indirect relationships to diet, and together they accounted for 247,000 cases in 1984.

Another way to understand the rates of cancer in affluent countries is to examine cases observed in migratory populations. For example, if we follow the statistics of people born of the same ethnic background in diverse parts of the world, we find that when they migrate to the United States their rate for certain types of cancer increases dramatically. A black émigré from Africa in the United States risks a rate of cancer approximately ten times that of his brother who stayed in Africa and maintained the African diet and way of life. The figures are similar for people who have emigrated from parts of the Orient, including Japan, and from other countries considered to be less developed. In the U.S. their cancer rate rises to the indigenous level, which is as much as ten times that of their native country.

Many studies have indicated that certain characteristics of our diet seem to predispose people toward cancer. These include the abundance of fat. Overweight people are more likely to get cancer. This includes people of all ages, but most of all it affects men and women of middle age, and it affects women more than men.

Another disorder typical of people at higher risk for certain cancers could be constipation. As we discussed in the chapter on fiber (Chapter 1), this doesn't mean that constipation causes cancer, but it is indicative of dietary patterns that may show a person is not eating many vegetables, fruits, or whole-grain foods. Studies show that people who regularly eat these kinds of foods may have a lower risk for certain kinds of cancer.

In a review of the relationship between diet and cancer, the National Research Council of the National Academy of Sciences recently published a report that implicated a lack of certain nutrients in cancer risk. Insufficient intakes of foods containing vitamin A and the carotenoids (precursors of vitamin A), vitamin C, dietary fiber, and the element selenium may place people at higher risk for cancer.

How Does Cancer Get Started?

The body's trillions of cells normally reproduce themselves in an orderly manner as tissue that is constantly renewed and replaced. For example, cells of the gastrointestinal tract are turned over approximately every few days; many bone cells are reproduced every 5 or 6 months and red blood cells every 120 days. Occasionally a cell undergoes an abnormal change and begins to proliferate uncontrollably. In this process of uncontrolled growth it no longer specifically resembles the tissue from which it got started but will form its own mass of cells, which we normally think of as a tumor. Some tumors are not necessarily cancerous at first, or they may be permanently benign, which means they don't necessarily spread or get any bigger. Other tumors are very cancerous even when very small.

Some experts postulate that we all have these "pretumors" forming regularly in our bodies. Usually they remain benign or even dissolve of their own accord. When one becomes malignant we call it cancer. As a cancerous tumor gets larger it starts to destroy normal tissue. At the beginning a tumor may be local, but as it proliferates, parts of it invade neighboring tissue and other organs.

Sometimes one of the cells becomes detached and gets carried by the blood system or the lymph system to another part of the body and it begins to grow there. This is called "metastasis." When metastasis occurs, the cancer is advanced and almost always fatal. Ultimately it destroys other tissue or it simply consumes the body's resources due to the rapid growth of cancer cells. Eventually the rest of the body wastes away.

When normal cells start to undergo nonspecific proliferation it is called the initiation phase of cancer. This initiation stage may be caused by a number of things. For example, certain types of radiation are initiators, literally altering the genetic makeup of the cells. Certain chemicals bring about the same result. So do certain viruses. And there is probably a heredity involvement in the initiation phase.

The second phase of cancer, the promotion phase, can take a long period of time, possibly ten or twenty years. In this prolonged phase, the growth of cells with the altered genetic material is influenced by its environment, including nutrients. A number of environmental factors seem to increase the growth of cells that have the potential to become cancerous. Among the tissues that have the greatest exposure to these factors are the lungs and the tissues of the alimentary canal. Lungs have a large surface area since they are like a myriad of small bubbles, and their environment contains the air we breathe. Smokers create an environment of harmful, irritating materials in their lungs regularly, and the more irritated the lungs, the more susceptible they are to cancer. The alimentary canal begins in the mouth and ends in the anus, including the digestive system. In nonsmokers these tissues have the greatest exposure to carcinogenic materials.

We can reduce the risk of cancer's developing in this long period. With regard to carcinogens such as radiation, smoke, and harmful chemicals, we can stay away from them as much as possible. Second, we can alter the diet, by removing components that promote cancer, and by adding dietary components that may protect the body cells from cancer initiators.

The High-Fiber-Food Connection

An example of a dietary protector is high-fiber food (Chapter 1), which moves material more quickly through the intestinal system and with a greater volume. If something in the diet promotes cancer, it will move through the system more quickly if the diet is high in fibrous foods. And since the volume of the stool is greater, the chemical will be less concentrated. Studies have shown that people who eliminate more frequently (such as vegetarians) generally have a lower incidence of certain types of cancer. In fact, the shorter bowel transit time of people living in Third World countries appears to make them less susceptible to certain cancers than residents of affluent countries, where the typical bowel transit time is often three days or more.

A low-fiber diet is usually higher in fat, and this combination may favor the development of a different microflora in the large intestine. A high-fiber diet seems to favor the development of a microflora that consists of more aerobic microorganisms (which grow in the presence of oxygen) than anaerobic microorganisms (which grow in the absence of oxygen). Some researchers believe that the microflora in a high-fiber diet is likely to be more protective.

Under certain conditions steroids produced by one's own liver and secreted into the intestinal tract can become carcinogenic. For example, in 1940 one of the by-products of steroid metabolism—one of the human bile acids—was found under some conditions to be weakly carcinogenic; constant exposure to it causes experimental animals to develop cancer. A diet that is high in fiber moves these fecal steroids through the system more quickly.

A high-fiber diet generally contains more fruits, vegetables, and grains—a diet associated with a lower rate of cancer. Studies indicate that there are other factors in these materials that may reduce the risk of cancer by providing various types of protection. These range from the indoles found in cruciferous vegetables (broccoli, Brussels sprouts, cauliflower, cabbage, kale, etc.) to vitamin C, which, as an antioxidant, prevents the conversion of nitrates to nitrosamines.

Fiber should be part of the food system throughout the day. A bowl of cereal in the morning is not enough. Fiber provides a matrix for everything going through the alimentary canal. It should especially be part of a meal rich in fat, for example processed meat or even steak.

The High-Fat Diet

Many studies done on cancer indicate that a diet high in dietary fat is more carcinogenic. Epidemiological evidence shows that a nation such as Japan with a low per capita intake of fat has a much lower incidence of and a much lower mortality from breast and colon cancer, for example, than a society that has a higher per capita consumption of fat, such as ours. The same seems to hold true for cancer of the prostate.

Precise mechanisms whereby dietary fat influences the carcinogenic process remain, to some extent, unknown. One theory put forth suggests that certain types of fat become rancid and it's the rancidity that causes the cancer. Another theory proposes that it's just fat in general and that more fat deposits lead to a greater deposit in the tissue of certain cancer-promoting agents.

Some researchers believe that polyunsaturated fats altered by high-temperature frying or by partial hydrogenation become part of the cell membrane and alter it, thus making it more permeable to cancer initiators. However, current research now underway should provide more evidence in the near future.

Salting, Smoking, and Pickling

A number of possible cancer-causing materials have been associated with cancer of the esophagus and cancer of the stomach. These are smoked, smoke-cured, salt-cured, or pickled foods, which have a high ability to irritate the esophagus and the stomach. It appears that for these agents to act as promoters of cancer they must be consumed regularly over a long period of time, as they are in such countries as Iceland, China, and Japan. With modernization of the diet, their consumption declines, as does the rate of cancer of the stomach and esophagus.

Effects of Vitamin C–Rich Foods

Nitrates and nitrites occur widely in the soil and in plants and can be converted in the digestive system to the nitrosamines, which are carcinogenic. When Popeye ate a great big serving of spinach to give him the strength to combat Bluto, he was also consuming some nitrates and nitrites in that spinach. (If the spinach was harvested on a cloudy rather than a sunny day, the nitrate level would have been higher.) In the stomach under a number of specific conditions such as high fat or excessive coffee consumption, nitrates and the nitrites can be converted to nitrosamines.

Dr. R. Raineri's laboratory experiments, which simulated the conditions of the human gastrointestinal tract, showed that vitamin C decreased the levels of nitrite and nitrosamine formation. This suggests that the conversion of nitrates and nitrites to nitrosamines may be inhibited when they are consumed with foods rich in vitamin C.

In plants where nitrates and nitrites occur, vitamin C is also available to prevent conversion to nitrosamines. In contrast, vitamin C is not naturally present when nitrates and nitrites are used in processed foods, especially cured meats, to inhibit the growth of the organisms that cause botulism, a deadly form of food poisoning. For a long time we did not realize that nitrates and nitrites could be converted to nitrosamines, especially in the presence of fat, which these cured meats so richly contain. Now that this process is known, it may be appropriate, if you choose to eat sausages or other preserved meats, to make sure you consume an adequate amount of vitamin C–rich foods at the same time.

A study by Dr. Sylvia Wassertheil-Smoller and others has associated low levels of dietary vitamin C with the possibility of developing cancer of the cervix. Some researchers analyzed the relationship between vitamin C intake and abnormal Papp smears and found a trend toward formation of precancerous cells in women who had low vitamin C intakes. This would not necessarily mean that low intake of vitamin C–rich foods causes cancer, but it does suggest that an adequate intake may help block the formation or effectiveness of a carcinogen.

Vitamin A to the Rescue

Several years ago epidemiologists found that people who consume a diet that yields ample vitamin A and the carotenoids (precursors of vitamin A) have a lower risk of cancer. This effect stands out most in smokers, who would be expected to be at highest risk, but even this elevated risk can be somewhat reduced by a diet rich in beta-carotene. However, as I've noted previously, no nutrient can completely undo the damage done by smoking.

When vitamin A is absent, tissue differentiation does not take place as effectively as it should and poor tissue growth can result. Conversely, adequate vitamin A helps to sustain normal cell differentiation. The precursor of vitamin A, beta-carotene, may itself protect against carcinogenic materials by serving as a type of antioxidant. Thus, it may protect the cell from the ravages of materials that seem to promote the formation of cancer.

Recent studies have shown an interrelationship between low beta-carotene intake and cancer of the uterus, which would indicate, once more, that this nutrient may act on cells as either an antioxidant or an antitumorigenic.

The evidence provided by these studies is not conclusive. Beta-carotene is not a necessary nutrient, nor can it conclusively be said to prevent cancer. But it seems apparent that a diet low in beta-carotene-rich foods predisposes an individual to certain types of cancer. Whether the culprit is lack of beta-carotene itself or some other factor in these foods remains to be determined.

Nevertheless the evidence for these correlations is so suggestive that the National Cancer Institute is conducting a study to test these effects of beta-carotene. In this study a large group of doctors will regularly consume a beta-carotene supplement for five years and their rate of cancer will be compared to that of a group that consumes a placebo (a supplement that looks like beta-carotene but isn't).

In light of current research findings, prudence dictates eating plenty of fruits and vegetables.

Vitamin E and Selenium

Vitamin E is a major antioxidant. It protects cells from oxidizing agents called free radicals, which can damage the cell by altering the cell membrane. Animal studies show that vitamin E protects polyunsaturated fatty acids from oxidation. It also seems to have a protective effect in humans, but the correlations are not conclusive.

Selenium has recently been identified as an essential trace element. Epidemiological studies have shown that as selenium becomes adequate in the diet the risk of cancer seems to decline. These findings indicate that a diet high in selenium-rich foods may be protective against certain types of cancer. Large quantities of selenium can be dangerous, however, so it's important to be cautious.

Overweight

Excessive body fat seems to be associated with the development of certain types of cancer. Breast cancer in women and prostate cancer in men involve organs that come under hormonal influence. One current theory postulates that obesity affects circulating levels of hormones, and hormones play an important role in influencing some cancers. Overweight people not only consume things that may help promote cancer, such as fat, but often fail to get enough dietary fiber and vitamins A and C. A high-fat diet is usually also high in empty calories, as opposed to calories from fruits, vegetables, and whole grains, which is where many of the preventive materials originate.

Folic Acid

Cancer involves alteration of the genetic material in the cell. In recent years some scientists have indicated that the susceptibility to alteration of this genetic material may be hereditary or the result of weakened genetic material. These weak points can be altered by radiation or through some type of cancer-causing chemical. These researchers have indicated that folic acid, a B vitamin (Chapter 6), which is essential in cell division, is also essential in making the weak points in genetic material stronger or repairing weak points when they occur. In fact, nature in her wisdom has a group of enzymes whose role is to repair DNA, the basic genetic material. Obviously, there will be much research devoted to these phenomena in the future. It's possible that folic acid plays a role in many of the enzymes and in the reproduction of the proteins that are used to protect the genetic material. Could it be that a person whose diet contains less than the recommended level of folic acid is more susceptible to the formation of cancer?

Alcohol

For years physicians have maintained that people with a high consumption of alcohol seem to be more susceptible to the development of certain types of cancer. They don't know whether it's the alcohol or (as people who drink excessively and then don't feel so good the next day always claim) other material in the alcoholic beverage. Suffice it to say that people who have a higher intake of alcohol, especially if they smoke or have a poor diet, are likely to have a higher incidence of cancer than people who do not. It's also known that people who have a high alcohol intake usually have a diet poor in a variety of other things, such as vitamin B and iron.

Nutritional Insurance

Since it is recognized that the diet may not be perfect, nutritional insurance with all the vitamins and minerals appears to be appropriate. In this chapter, we have identified possible roles for foods rich in vitamin A, vitamin C, and selenium. A person can develop a plan of nutritional health insurance to make sure that he gets the recommended daily allowance of every single vitamin and mineral that is recognized by science. It can be done by the simple use of supplements that contain the nutrients in a balanced appropriate quantity. But there is no evidence that taking nutrients above the RDA will prevent cancer. For instance, excessive amounts of vitamins A and D can be toxic (see Chapters 2 and 3). Fiber and beta-carotene intakes should also be adequate.

Recent studies have indicated that men who exercise regularly are less likely to get colon cancer. This doesn't teach us anything we didn't know—a balanced diet, fresh air, and exercise are necessary for good health. With regard to cancer, we can also add some other advice: don't smoke, don't drink excessively, maintain ideal weight, avoid exposure to harmful chemicals, pollutants, and excessive sunlight. In short, practice the sage old advice: "moderation in all things."

Nutrition and Disease: Changing Concepts

PETER V. SACKS, M.D.

What is a fatal disease? If you had asked that of someone
fifty years ago, they would have replied smallpox, diphtheria,
or tuberculosis. Yet these are diseases we hardly think about
today. Why? Because modern science developed vaccines and
antibiotics to protect us from these scourges. Ask someone
today to name a fatal disease and odds are they'll say cancer.
If not cancer, then heart disease, high blood pressure, or
stroke. The difference? The killer diseases of yore stemmed
from infectious bacteria. They would invade a susceptible
host, and within a few hours or days the unfortunate person
knew he was ill. Today's killers build slowly over a lifetime.
Each fatty meal, each day without exercise, each exposure to
pollutants adds just a little bit more damage until enough
accumulates to cause heart disease, cancer, or a stroke. These
diseases are not infectious. You do not catch them from
someone else. They are what we call lifestyle diseases,
encompassing a cluster of factors, prime among them
nutrients of which we get too much, such as fat, or too little,
such as fiber and beta-carotene.

What is malnutrition? Up until very recently, anyone
would have said undernourishment, not getting enough to eat.
Images of starving populations in Third World nations would
inevitably come to mind. Today, however, we take the term
more literally. We have come to recognize that obesity, a
major health problem in affluent societies, can be a form of

malnutrition. Just as the starving person's lack of nutritious food is detrimental to his health, the obese person's overconsumption of food, especially nonnutritious food, is hazardous to his.

What is a nutritional deficiency? Just a few years ago we would have defined it as the lack of a dietary element, especially a vitamin or mineral, that emerges as specific symptoms in a matter of months. But today we know that a lack of fiber in the diet may go undetected for years—thirty-year-olds seldom develop diverticulosis or colon cancer. Fiber is not a vitamin or mineral and there are no established dietary requirements as yet. All the same, a fiber deficiency, a result of the refining of our food supply, seems to appear with specific symptoms. In a slightly different vein, classic deficiency symptoms for various vitamins and minerals we call "antioxidants" are hard to find in our society. Yet evidence indicates that these substances may exert a protective effect against cancer. What then constitutes a deficiency?

New discoveries of recent decades are changing our fundamental concepts about disease, malnutrition, and nutritional deficiencies. We now realize that good nutrition is more than the absence of scurvy and the other classic deficiency diseases. Good nutrition also means the absence of obesity, gout, high blood pressure, heart disease, and certain types of cancer. Good nutrition is preventive medicine; they are indivisible. That recognition and the implementation of all it implies may be as big a breakthrough for health in our era as defeating bacteria was for generations in the past. There is every reason to believe that, as discoveries continue, cancer and heart disease will be as rare to future generations as smallpox and diphtheria are to us.

14

HOW ALL THIS
CAME TO PASS
Taste and Survival

We humans are omnivores. We eat fruits, vegetables, grains, meat, dairy products, fish, and other foods. Within these broad categories, diets vary widely. A tribe in the jungles of South America lives almost exclusively on fermented grain products; the mainstay of their diet is a kind of beer. A tribe in Africa raise cattle but, in addition to drinking the milk, they extract blood, which is the staple of their diet.

Human beings require many nutrients, and variety makes it possible for us to get everything we need. Throughout history we have had to supplement our basic diet to obtain sufficient amounts of essential nutrients. As these chapters show, our ingenuity has made it all possible.

The Optimal Diet

We consume about a pound in dry weight of food per day. Of this, macrominerals, such as calcium, phosphorus, sodium, and potassium, amount to several grams, and about another gram consists of vitamins and other minerals.

We obtain three macronutrients (four counting fiber) from our diet—protein, fat, and carbohydrates. Each one is important in the correct proportion. Nutritionists have developed what is generally accepted as the prudent or optimal diet. Assuming all other nutritional requirements are met, an optimal diet will promote excellent health by the judicious juxtaposition of protein, fat, and carbohydrates.

The optimal diet would contain 10 to 12 percent of its calories as protein (which provides four calories per gram) and 30 percent or fewer of its calories from fat (which yields nine calories per gram). As stated in Chapter 12, the amounts of saturated and polyunsaturated fats should be approximately equal. (Another class of fats, the monounsaturated fats, high in such foods as olive oil, are considered to be neutral to health.) Fifty-eight to 60 percent of calories should come from carbohydrates (which like protein provide four calories per gram).

An optimal diet of 2,000 calories per day, more than most women consume, would contain approximately 220 calories or 55 grams of protein, 600 calories or 67 grams of fat, and 1,180 calories or approximately 295 grams of carbohydrates. That totals only 417 grams, which is somewhat under a pound, not including fiber, which is not digested and should be at least 25 grams and preferably up to 50 grams.

Protein

In a diet that contains meat, fish, poultry, milk (or other dairy products), and eggs, adequate protein is not an issue. In contrast, a strict vegetarian diet requires a careful balance of grains, legumes, mushrooms, and other vegetables in order to get the right combination of amino acids needed for complete protein.

Protein supplements are helpful in obtaining sufficient protein of high quality without the fat content of meat and dairy products. Often, these supplements are from vegetable sources, which shows that proper combination is all that's necessary to obtain adequate protein without eating animal products.

Fat

Fat consists of saturated fat, which is hard at room temperature like the white marbling in and around meat, and unsaturated fat, which is liquid at room temperature. Unsaturated fat consists of polyunsaturated fat (PUFA), which is light, such as corn oil, or monounsaturated, which is heavier, as found in large quantities in olive oil. For polyunsaturated fat to be made hard like margarine it must be made more saturated by a process known as hydrogenation.

An optimal diet restricts fat to 30 percent of total calories and controls the saturated fat from meat to less than about 10 percent of calories, balanced by an equal or greater amount of PUFA. The remainder, monounsaturated fat, is considered neutral from a health standpoint.

Carbohydrates

Carbohydrates come in two forms, simple and complex. Simple carbohydrates generally consist of table sugar (sucrose), the fruit sugars (glucose and fructose), and milk sugar (lactose). Complex carbohydrates consist of the starches found in cereals, grains, vegetables, legumes, and some fruits. These can be processed into a wide variety of food products.

A prudent diet will strive for at least half of its carbohydrate calories in the complex form, and as much of the simple carbohydrates as possible from fruits and vegetables, rather than table sugar made from cane or sugar beets.

The Two Faces of Malnutrition

When you say "malnutrition" the average American thinks of a child with a bloated stomach, barely enough flesh to cover his bones, and flies crawling over his face.

But, with all its terrible truth, this image distracts from a less visible but equally distressing situation. If we could suddenly feed every one of those children on the verge of starvation, we'd only be scratching the surface of malnutrition. A less extreme, less noticeable, but infinitely more widespread form of malnutrition also has a great impact on the welfare of the world's people. It is the malnutrition of those who are just getting by, not quite sick enough to merit attention or relief, but caught in a self-perpetuating cycle of suboptimal mental and physical development that holds whole societies down for generation after generation.

Even more scandalous—because it's totally unnecessary —is the malnutrition of those who are literally killing themselves with the diet of affluence. Like the malnutrition of poverty, the malnutrition of overprocessed food and overweight demands greater scrutiny from government, educational institutions, and industry.

Reaching the Genetic Potential

From the moment of conception, every human being is endowed with a physiological potential as to physical growth, mental development, resistance to disease, and longevity. Fulfillment of this potential is often discussed in terms of shelter, education, medicine, and the social environment. But the overriding factor is food. More than any other influence, the quality of a person's diet, especially in the prenatal months and early childhood, determines whether his potential will be achieved—and perhaps extended beyond the limits we accept today—or permanently stifled.

To appreciate fully the role of nutrition in realizing human potential, we must examine affluent and nonaffluent people. For the purposes of this discussion, affluence does not denote geopolitical boundaries or socio-economic groups, but access to an optimal diet.

The affluent person is able to obtain at least as many calories as he must expend to function productively. There is enough variety in his diet to ensure sufficient protein of adequate quality and the necessary amounts of vitamins and minerals. His nutritional problems are likely to be those of excess calories, especially in the form of fat and sugar.

The nonaffluent person cannot always obtain enough calories to satisfy the energy requirements of a normal day's activity. His protein intake is inadequate, and what he does get is often of poor quality, thus restricting his physiological growth and development. With a limited variety of foods available to him, he is likely to be deficient in some vitamins and minerals.

By far the most important factor is protein, made up of amino acids, which are the building blocks of tissue growth and replacement. Of some twenty-two amino acids, all but eight are synthesized by the adult body. It is the extent to which they are all present in the correct proportion that determines whether dietary protein is of high or low quality.

The essential amino acids are most readily available through the meat, fish, poultry, and dairy products that abound in the diet of the affluent, where protein provides at least 10 to 15 percent of calorie intake, with 40 to 45 percent coming from fat and the remaining 40 to 50 percent from carbohydrates. By contrast, the nonaffluent person derives about 80 percent of his calories from carbohydrates. The plant protein inherent in a high-carbohydrate diet offers far less in terms of both quantity and quality than the animal protein in a high-fat diet. In fact, without proper complementation, very often the grain foods that characterize the nonaffluent diet are not sufficient, by themselves, to support adequate growth.

For every case of kwashiorkor or marasmus, the diseases of extreme protein or calorie deficiency that afflict infants, there are unknown hundreds of children who are malnourished but unnoticed because they show none of the obvious signs of deterioration. These members of the nonaffluent population have a smaller body size than the affluent. Traditionally this difference was attributed to genetics.

That kind of thinking went out the window when dietary improvements started turning out a generation of tall Japanese and Taiwanese. It is well known that the key to growth of tissue and bone is not exclusively the province of some set of ethnic genes, but also depends on adequate calories, vitamins, and minerals, (especially calcium) available in the diet.

Strong circumstantial evidence associates protein malnutrition during the fetal period and the first three years of life with underdeveloped mental capacity. Severely malnourished babies, especially those with low birth weight, have smaller brains with fewer cells than those of well-nourished children. They lag behind in intellectual performance and, unfortunately, many studies suggest that they will never catch up no matter how much their diets may improve after age three.

In contrast, consider children who were well nourished as infants, but suffered severe deprivation from age three to six. This happened to many children during World War II. After returning to an adequate diet they were able to reestablish mental parity with children who had suffered no malnutrition.

Resistance to Disease

To children in affluent populations, childhood diseases are usually little more than a nuisance. Among the nonaffluent, they can kill. We can only guess at how many millions of deaths they actually cause, because census figures on infant mortality are incomplete. In some places, children are given such a small chance of survival that they aren't even counted as "births" until they reach the age of two. It is estimated that fewer children born in nonaffluent groups reach age five, compared to the number of children among the affluent.

Infectious diseases are generally precipitated by unsanitary conditions and easily spread among dense populations, but the body's ability to resist them is clearly a function of nutrition. The antibodies that fight infection are elaborate protein systems. Without adequate dietary protein, the body can neither resist disease nor repair tissues that are damaged as a result. A downward spiral is set in motion: as the body's defenses are overtaxed, malnourishment becomes more severe, and malnutritional diarrhea results in dehydration and further loss of nutrients. This, in turn, further decreases resistance to disease, often leading to death.

Malnutrition Among the Affluent

Life expectancy at birth among the affluent increased from forty-seven years in 1900 to seventy-three years in 1980, an increase of nearly 50 percent. But life expectancy at age sixty-five increased by less than 23 percent in the same eight decades, from

11.9 to 14.6. Throughout history, since Biblical times, people have speculated on how long humans can live. We don't know. It's a matter of heredity, diet, and lifestyle.

Death comes to the affluent from three major causes: cardiovascular disease (52 percent); cancer (25 percent); accidents, suicide, and homicide (8 percent); and diabetes, liver, and kidney diseases (4 percent). That accounts for almost 90 percent of all deaths. In most of these fatalities nutrition is a very important—often the predominant—factor. The average "well-fed" man will die in his sixties or seventies (often earlier) *not* because it is the natural time for his body to fail him, but because he's been eating the wrong things all his life. With 60 percent of deaths related to what could be dietary management, it's obvious that life could be prolonged to achieve the full measure of an individual's genetic lifespan, typically 90 to 100 years.

Cardiovascular disease (CVD) broadly encompasses many disorders of the heart and circulatory system. Heart disease caused by atherosclerosis—the deposition of a fatty substance called plaque on arterial walls—is the predominant form of CVD. The accumulation of plaque, which in sufficient quantities can cause arterial blockages that result in heart attack, is associated with the level of serum cholesterol in the blood. Cardiovascular diseases involving deposits on arterial walls also can result in stroke, which accounts for 11 percent of all deaths among the affluent.

The precise causes of heart disease cannot be pinned down, though, because so many other factors are involved, usually in combination with each other. Hereditary susceptibility, body weight, physical inactivity, cigarette smoking, high blood cholesterol levels, and high blood pressure are among the indicators we call "risk factors."

It is clear, though, that most of these factors are diet related. The person who is overweight, thereby running a risk of heart attack two or three times greater than someone of average weight, simply eats more calories than he burns up. Physical inactivity, which produces similarly high odds of an attack, may be the product not only of a sedentary occupation but of a cyclic effect, in which the burden of added weight discourages exercise, which leads to further weight gain, and so on.

Someone with a systolic blood pressure above 160 may double or triple his chances of heart attack. A high diastolic blood pressure may also be risky. Although genetics is one of the major determinants of high blood pressure, its origins are thought to be dietary in a large percentage of cases. Many of them may be controlled by restriction of salt intake.

The blood cholesterol reading is a key indicator, because it relates to the all-important balance between saturated and polyunsaturated fats in our diet, as well as dietary cholesterol. Cholesterol counts tell us that far too many members of the affluent population are courting disaster with their carnivorous ways. There is a widespread need to reduce the intake of saturated fats (primary sources of which are meat and dairy products) and increase consumption of the polyunsaturated fats (which abound in various vegetable oils).

About 30 percent of all cancer deaths involve the alimentary-excretory systems. Science is bringing to the fore a number of dietary factors that can at least reduce the probability of getting cancer (Chapter 13).

Productivity and Precedent

Who can measure the cost when people from forty to sixty-five, the years when all their education and experience culminate in peaks of productivity and responsibility, become seriously ill? What are the social and economic costs—to the individuals, to their employers, to the entire society—of their failure to maintain balanced, healthy diets? No one can attach a numerical answer to these questions, but the list of long-term illnesses that are related to the malnutrition of the affluent is staggering: cardiovascular disease, obesity, and colonic cancers get the most attention, but diet is often involved in anemia, diverticular disease, hypertension, diabetes, liver disease, mental illness, skin problems, and osteoporosis.

The affluent diet is too rich in calories, fat, and sugar, and that trend is set in early childhood. The causes of heart disease don't suddenly begin in middle age; it just takes that long to notice them. Plaque deposits may start building up in early adolescence. The consequences of childhood excesses are not technically irreversible—unlike the permanent damage suffered by deprived nonaffluent infants—but our lack of attention to the problem means it's unlikely to be corrected.

In this context I will examine dietary development.

Lines of Defense

Before considering the twentieth century, think of primitive man and the basic tools he used to identify foods that would provide safe sustenance. The first line of defense in selecting foods is smell, which often allows us to detect things that have decayed, are rotten, or would otherwise be unsafe to consume. When certain foods rot or are spoiled by bacteria, obnoxious by-products arc given off. These range from complex materials such as putrescine to simple gases such as hydrogen sulfide. Our olfactory system is capable of detecting very small quantities of these by-products. For example, we can detect hydrogen sulfide in parts per billion.

Our second line of defense is taste. Certain taste buds help us detect and ward off food problems. At birth, we are already capable of detecting sweet, bitter, and salty. In nature, sweet food is relatively safe and good for us—good because it provides calories. For example, fruits are sweet; they contain lots of carbohydrates, which provide energy and are safe. A soldier is taught that to survive in the wilds he should eat only natural things that are sweet if he doesn't recognize them as safe. Sweet foods usually also have a pleasant odor. For example, smell is used by knowledgeable people to select a ripe melon.

We are also born with the ability to detect bitter and sour. Foods that are bitter are usually unsafe to eat. Acorns are an example. How our forefathers discovered the technique of rendering acorns edible by boiling and filtering them is lost in antiquity, but in this process the bitterness disappears. Similarly with the roots of certain plants, some of which are Third World staples.

We are also born with the capability of detecting saltiness. In primitive times the ability to avoid salty or brackish water was essential, since pure, fresh water is the most essential nutrient next to air itself.

Cultivated Tastes

In the last part of the twentieth century we have cultivated a taste for salty food even though we would not think of drinking salt water. At one time salt was so scarce that people were literally paid in salt and the word "salary" comes directly from it (Chapter 11). Now that salt is nearly free, we use prodigious amounts, especially in prepared foods. Some simple statistics will make the point. Soup mixes are often 20 percent salt by weight. Chicken, which usually has less than 100 milligrams of salt per serving (say a breast) contains about 900 milligrams or more as it is served in a fast-food outlet. Processed cereals usually have salt as one of their first three ingredients.

A desire for a texture, considered by some a taste, is the desire for fat. This craving for fat had survival value for our primitive ancestors, who needed to sock away extra calories in between successful hunts. Today the only thing we have to hunt for is a parking space at the supermarket or restaurant, where we indulge that fat craving to unhealthy extremes.

Other Lines of Defense

Toxic materials often cause vomiting, which is another natural way of eliminating bad components from the diet. Indeed, one approach to first-aid in poisoning is to induce vomiting. The stomach also produces copious quantities of acid, which in the course of digestion can kill some microorganisms that would otherwise cause health problems.

The final line of defense is the liver. Anatomically the first stop that most digested materials make on their way throughout the body, the liver, is where certain materials are detoxified. For example, alcohol, a toxic material, is rendered neutral in the liver when consumed in moderation, and converted to energy. Unfortunately, excess alcohol intake may lead to cirrhosis of the liver, one cause of death in this country.

The Evolution of Cuisine

Most food systems developed around the question of how to produce sufficient protein despite a scarcity of meat and of ways to preserve the meat that was available.

For example, French cuisine is known for its rich sauces and elaborate preparation; in fact, many ethnic dishes of Europe are prepared in this way. Creative impetus for this type of food may have come from the need to use meat of questionable quality and in limited amounts. Horse was often the only meat available. In fact, gelatin was developed during sieges that forced cooks to use even the bones, hooves, and hides for food. Sauces were made with the meat drippings, which provide many vitamins.

Another way to disguise meat of dubious quality and also to make small amounts go a long way is to add curry powder. The spices used sometimes helped to prevent spoilage and inhibit microorganism growth.

Many Asian cuisines use meat as a condiment. As a condiment, it raises the total quality of protein in the meal. People who cook with a wok can take a chicken breast, slice it into very small pieces, stir-fry it with vegetables, and have a meal for a family of four, whereas an average family of four would need four chicken breasts, either barbecued or broiled. The high percentage of fiber (as discussed in Chapter 1) in the large amount of vegetables provides a great deal of bulk and helps make the meal satisfying.

Wok cooking evolved at a time when fuel was in short supply and often consisted of dried animal droppings. A small amount of oil is heated to a very high temperature with a minimum of fuel and, in this manner, thin strips or cubes of vegetables, meat, poultry, or fish can be cooked very quickly. A small volume of material is immersed briefly in the oil, and as the cooked material is pushed up the sides of the wok, oil is allowed to drain back into the center so it can be used to cook other things. The short cooking time also preserves the vitamins.

Pasta

Pasta, the Italian staple, is a means of preserving wheat. In the form of pasta, grain keeps for a long time and provides adequate protein and complex carbohydrates. However, it doesn't provide much taste. With an interesting sauce, especially based upon tomatoes, pasta allows a small amount of meat and cheese to go a very long way. At the same time, this diet keeps the fat to a minimum, and the use of cheese, especially low-fat cheese like mozzarella or ricotta, provides calcium and protein, again without too much fat.

Safety

Many exotic international cuisines consist of hot, spicy meals and contain components that some twentieth-century Americans regard as very difficult to eat, such as garlic, hot spices, and peppers. The usual joke or cartoon portrays a person eating this food and flames coming out of his mouth. Think of Mexican or Szechuan cuisine or Indian curries. In these hotter climates, parasites abound that can lead to dysentery and other illness. Perhaps, some of the causative organisms may be killed by the various spices, peppers, and condiments.

In Chapter 12 we saw that garlic has antibiotic-like properties. Also other components, such as various types of Mexican peppers, may be capable of rendering many of these microorganisms harmless or killing them; consequently, this is a way of providing more safety in a simple, natural dietary system. A good illustration is the *turista*, a diarrhea contracted by drinking water or eating salads contaminated with certain microorganisms. If tourists would eat only native food that is well cooked and contains hot peppers and spices that may have the ability to destroy these organisms, they would be more likely to come out unscathed if their palates could survive.

Gross Affluence

As a people of plenty in a temperate climate, Americans have not had to use meat as a condiment or to use strong spices to preserve it or sauces to conceal failures of preservation. In Europe it was a sign of wealth to eat lots of meat, not lots of vegetables; symbolic of this was the feudal lord with his large roasts and plentiful bounty of game. As our capacity to produce evolved in the U.S. the capacity to serve meat was democratized. Americans ate enormous quantities of meat, especially steaks and roasts. Processed sausage meats with their high fat content became delicacies that technology made available to all.

The introduction of food technology around the turn of the century started to make available to us large quantities of highly processed flour, which allowed us to eat things that normally would be available only to the rich. This introduction of technology focused on grains and cereals and started to remove fiber from the diet. Fiber was replaced with fat, salt, and sugar, which are the primary ingredients available to the food technologists in addition to water and air.

We have also focused on sweetness. As sugar became readily available, per capita consumption went from about 70 pounds of sugar annually at the turn of the century to the current total of about 130 pounds annually. Most of this sugar is found in the various processed foods we consume, and sweetness has now become one of the expected sensations. For example, the introduction of the carbonated soft beverage has brought a decline in consumption of milk and dairy products. With this shift, the ever-continuing problem of obtaining enough calcium was intensified. As a result billions will be spent on joint prosthetic surgery, much of which is the result of brittle bones (see Chapter 7).

Learning What We Want

A major vector in the food business is advertising, which can create a need for things that serve no purpose other than pleasure. An analysis of advertising expenditures related to food shows that approximately 86 percent is devoted to foods that contain nothing more than empty calories and are not wholesome by many standards. Examples include soft drinks, candies, and cereals that provide little more than simple sugar. In fact, the advertising expenditures for two major soft drinks exceed the government budget (in USDA) devoted to nutrition education.

The twentieth century could be called the "fat" century, as fat has emerged as the texture of preference. This is most obviously recognized in the increase of fast-food outlets that mostly sell meat—meat in its simplified, almost homogenized form, the all-American hamburger. In outlets that sell chicken, fish, or low-fat foods, the central ingredients are deep-fat fried and then a sauce is added, both of which add more fat to the meal. In many of these fast-food outlets over 50 percent of the calories are usually derived from fat, even in chicken dishes. At the same time, the vegetable, which was the central portion of many cuisines, has become the garnish in our society. This is a flaunting of affluence.

Along with this rise in meat consumption is a decline in organ-meat consumption and an increase in processed meats, such as frankfurters and foods that provide a major percentage of their calories as fat with very few redeeming features.

What Can We Do?

We can examine our diet and recover control over what we eat. Examine the distribution of your calories and ask, "Am I malnourished?" If the answer is yes, make some fundamental changes. A few rules can start you on your way:

- Only one meal with meat, fish, or poultry each day; vegetarians could use some dairy products, eggs, beans, and some grains.

- Two pieces of fruit each day.
- Several servings of vegetables, grains, beans each day.
- Dairy products each day.
- Alcohol in moderation, not more than twice a week.
- Dessert at only one meal.
- Never use a salt shaker.

15

GRANDMOTHER WASN'T ALWAYS RIGHT
Nutritional Fallacies

When it comes to food, old wives' tales often have sound nutrition principles behind them. Because of these handed-down homilies, supplementation of the diet has existed for thousands of years, long before scientists isolated and identified vitamins in their laboratories, in fact long before there were scientists and laboratories.

Granted, the old methods of supplementation were a far cry from the tablets and capsules of today, but they were often just as effective. Bringing children out into the January sun is not as convenient as giving them a tablet containing vitamin D. Pushing nails through an apple, allowing it to sit, removing the nails and eating the apple is not as easy as taking iron tablets after a doctor tells you that you're anemic. Brewing tea from pine needles or rose hips during the winter months is not as fast as popping a vitamin C tablet. In each case, however, the goal and results are the same.

Since women were the ones who traditionally stocked the family pantry, planned the meals, and tended the sick, it's little wonder that they were the ones to discover and pass on good advice. An apple a day kept the doctor away—and a rhyme or catchy phrase helped the next generation remember what grandma always used to say.

However, grandmother wasn't always right, nor was mother for that matter. Our cultural lore contains much fine-sounding advice that actually can do more harm than good. For example, the biggest health problem our society now faces is overweight, which is implicated in diabetes, hypertension, heart disease, and possibly cancer. Yet much well-intended folklore encourages children to eat more than their appetites indicate is necessary.

These admonitions may cause emotional eating disorders for life, ranging all the way from compulsive eating to compulsive starving (as in anorexia nervosa). It can also lead to a combination of the two as in bulimia, a pattern of gorging and then vomiting up the food. These eating disorders have become serious health problems, particularly for young American women.

When a parent tells a child to "clear your plate today so we'll have a clear day tomorrow," the child may learn to eat everything that's served, but the lesson is not necessarily wise or even safe. Unfortunately, a loving but misguided parent may heap the child's plate with adult-size portions that far exceed the child's actual caloric needs. Usually, children eat enough to achieve a healthy energy balance without anyone's forcing them or, worse yet, attaching mystical or emotional significance to eating excess food.

"What a good eater he is!" (or she is!) a proud grandmother, grandfather, or parent will exclaim as food is shoveled into a tot's mouth. The child can't help but notice all the pleasure and excitement generated. If praise doesn't work, some parents will try guilt: "Think of the starving children in India." Or Africa. Or somewhere. They imply that finishing all of the mashed potatoes or peas will somehow prevent other children from starving. What this does is establish an eating pattern that overcomes the child's inborn appetite regulator. Better to instruct a child not to accept more food on his plate than he or she can eat and make second helpings available.

Obviously, a child needs to consume an adequate diet to support growth and maintain optimal health. But this can be encouraged by commending the child calmly for eating, as we would for displaying good table manners.

Obviously, too much emphasis on eating can lead to overweight, particularly in later years when physical growth tapers off, requiring less food and energy. Then the person so persuasively rewarded for overeating will receive a different message from the same concerned people, such as, "You need to lose weight. Stop eating so much."

How many overweight people "reward" themselves for all kinds of things with a rich, sweet dessert? "Finish those string beans and you'll get some ice cream," they recall mother or grandmother saying. In the words of a popular commercial, "You deserve a break today." The underlying idea is that we all lead such difficult lives that we are entitled to every pleasure we desire. But how often are we told we owe it to ourselves to lead a long, healthy life free from the hazards of overweight? Early food training may lead not only to overweight but to superstitions about eating, in the form of either unnecessary aversions or unwarranted attractions. For example, athletes often regard certain foods or dietary practices as almost sacred. If he or she eats a certain food before competing in an athletic event and performs well, the athlete may associate that food with superior performance. Certainly diet is important in athletic performance—entire books are written on the subject. However, once a diet is balanced, minor food changes have little to do with performance. The key factor is training, clear and simple. Sound nutrition is part of long-term training, not simply a single one-meal event. Superstitions about the effects of food on performance abound in all areas of life.

Scientific Illiteracy and Nutritional Quackery

A society that does not emphasize training in science during elementary and secondary school years should not be surprised when many of its members are unable to distinguish between legitimate science and pseudo-science.

In the U.S., for example, science and math scores on standardized college entrance exams have dropped steadily over the last twenty years. During elementary-school years, many American students probably get at most forty-five minutes of math and twenty minutes of science on a daily basis. Many schools do not introduce science until junior high school, and of all high school graduates who have completed three years of math, only a fifth have taken three years of science courses; less than 10 percent have studied physics. This problem is compounded by the lack of qualified science and math teachers for secondary schools.

Why should we be concerned with this in a book on nutrition? Without a grasp of basic scientific principles an individual is easy prey for quackery and fraud, which are not unknown in the area of nutrition and nutrition supplementation.

Americans are very concerned about their health, yet most know more about the workings of a car engine than they do about the workings of their own bodies. Bogus claims made by a pseudo-scientist may sound just as reasonable as the results of the most tightly controlled clinical study. Scientific illiterates crave simple answers to complex health-related issues. Thus, they are more likely to embrace the "works-overnight" cures of charlatans than the complex findings that emerge from our nation's top universities and research hospitals.

Anecdotal claims bombard us. Sometimes they lead to great discoveries, such as a scientist wanting to know why people who eat—or don't eat—certain foods avoid certain diseases. Personal anecdotes about health have often proved the starting point for exhaustive research. In legitimate science, however, mere anecdote is never enough; for pseudo-science it is often regarded as sufficient.

Many of the nutritional concepts explored in this book started as anecdotal claims, but they have stood the test of both extensive observation and the controlled experiments of science. The methods people used to supplement their diets were developed through trial and error over generations to bring about positive results that helped make possible the health of certain societies.

As scientific methods and instruments evolved, most of these folkloric nutrition practices underwent intensive scientific scrutiny. Even today, as we saw most recently with the Greenland Eskimos and the fish oil called EPA, they are tested and retested. They usually prove as solid as Gibraltar. Why bother testing them? To find out exactly what it is in a particular food that is beneficial to health, how much is needed for it to be effective, for how long and under what conditions it should be eaten.

Many health-related anecdotal claims we hear today lack the support of scientific research. Yet, to those who don't know otherwise, they may be more persuasive than scientific fact.

Part of this is due to the way the information is routinely presented. Solid data from a prestigious scientific institution are seldom presented with the same razzle-dazzle as a pseudo-scientific "discovery." The former is usually difficult to read. It is full of terms that are hard for the nonscientist to understand and full of qualifying statements that make it accurate but tedious. Thus legitimate science often lacks the show-biz impact of pseudoscience and is likely to be ignored by the scientifically illiterate.

To add insult to injury, entire publications exist to report "astounding new scientific breakthroughs." But a careful reader finds that the articles, if they refer to data at all, cite studies done in some obscure clinic in Hungary or some other far-off place, without the statistics available for evaluation. "Studies" such as this are never published in the journals of the scientific community and thus are unavailable to be checked by serious researchers. These "breakthroughs" simply can't meet the most basic standards of scientific investigation.

What's the harm? These unsubstantiated "breakthroughs" often become the basis for nutritional quackery. People begin diagnosing potentially dangerous illnesses themselves and using vitamins and minerals as drugs. Sometimes they urge others to take exceptionally high levels of vitamins and minerals. At these levels the nutrients are no longer comparable to what you would find in foods.

In the last several decades especially, various naturally occurring chemicals have been put forth as cancer cures, heart-disease cures, and aids to increasing physical energy. Unfortunately, most people don't know enough about science to assess these substances intelligently. Otherwise the promotions would fade away and people would save their money.

Nutrition's realm is the same as it always has been since early humans first evolved rituals for eating organ meats: the maintenance of optimum health and the prevention of disease. Curing disease is the responsibility of medicine. Unfortunately, the abuse of food supplements by pseudo-scientists endangers people's lives and gives nutrition a bad name.

Overdoses and Safety

The benefits of sensible nutrition have been described for millennia—there's even a reference in the Book of Daniel in the Old Testament. But megadosing is new to our era. When vitamin A was consumed in the form of beef liver, it was difficult to overdose. The same is true of vitamin D derived from sunshine. But with access to bottles of vitamin pills we can easily ingest as much as we like. For some reason, perhaps the good reputation of the name "vitamin," people today think that if a little is good, more is better. But taking much greater amounts than the body was designed to handle can be dangerous.

Safety is a serious concern in the case of the fat-soluble vitamins, A and D. With water-soluble vitamins the body can excrete excess amounts, but these fat-soluble vitamins are stored in the liver and other tissues. For example, a person ingesting ten times the RDA of vitamins A and D for prolonged periods of time may accumulate toxic levels. The annals of medicine provide examples of such excesses. In fact, these problems sometimes occur when physicians prescribe a vitamin to clear up a specific problem and the patient continues taking the vitamin at the therapeutic level after the recommended time is up. More frequently, a consumer just buys a pill that boasts 1000 percent of the RDA because he or she thinks it's better than 100 percent.

Because the body turns over 25 to 75 percent of the water-soluble B vitamins daily, it's often assumed that taking excessive amounts is not harmful, on the theory that the body simply excretes whatever it doesn't need. But even here recent evidence points out that the body cannot tolerate vast extremes. Scientific journals reported isolated cases of several women who took more than 250 times the RDA of vitamin B_6 for several months. The result: neurological damage. So even certain water-soluble vitamins appear to have safety limits. In addition, some scientists are concerned that taking single B-vitamin supplements in unbalanced amounts can cause metabolic imbalance as they may trigger excretion of other B vitamins.

Vitamin C, another water-soluble vitamin, is also cause for concern in individuals genetically predisposed to kidney-stone formation. Although scientists are debating the RDA itself, most agree that taking six grams or more per day may be unhealthy. Excess vitamin C intake creates a metabolic by-product called oxalic acid, which may lead to kidney stones in some genetically predisposed individuals.

Nor can we exonerate minerals from safety concerns. For example, zinc taken in doses ten times the RDA seems to cause a shift in blood cholesterol from the good type (HDL) to the bad type (LDL). This kind of excess also interferes with copper absorption, possibly leading to copper deficiency.

Everything, it seems, is harmful in excess. For example, water is essential to life but you can drown in it. Sunshine is beneficial but too much can give you sunburn and possibly skin cancer. Likewise, although the body needs nutrients, every mineral, it seems, can be harmful if taken in large enough quantities for a prolonged period of time. Back in the days when people supplemented their diets with iron by sticking nails in an apple, safety was not a concern. But with the ready availability of supplements excessive doses are easy to come by.

The concern for safety has to be considered for newer types of supplements as well, especially if there is no RDA to use as a yardstick. For example, a few capsules of EPA provide no more of this fatty acid than eating a serving of fresh salmon each day. Well-documented scientific evidence suggests that the health benefits make it worth doing. But, again, more is not better. We do not yet know of any toxic effects of excess EPA but that does not mean that none exist.

The watchword for safety is common sense. Examine supplement labels carefully, with moderation and balance as your guides. Evaluate the credentials of the promoter and his or her vested interest. Ask for information on safety and efficacy and don't accept personal anecdotes or allusions to a sole research project done by some obscure institution. After all, some of the world's greatest universities and hospitals are seldom more than a few hours' drive from your door. Know the RDAs. By definition, RDAs are "the levels of intake of essential nutrients considered in the judgment of the Food and Nutrition Board (National Academy of Sciences), on the basis of available scientific knowledge, to be adequate to meet the known nutritional needs of practically all healthy persons." Keep in mind that scientific knowledge is constantly changing, and so with it the scientific consensus. That's why the RDAs are revised approximately every five years. A nutrient level that may be considered high today could be the RDA of the future (see table, pp. 194–195).

The Future

Supplementation is now in a new era, making it possible to separate our food from our nutrition. Engineering makes it possible to formulate any combination of nutrients in many forms.

Science and technology now permit us to examine our health in great detail, evaluate our food with equal precision, and take supplements to remedy any dietary shortfalls, thus making available to everyone the opportunity to achieve optimum health. From grappling with scurvy, nutrition science has now advanced to the fine tuning of the body involved with blood-platelet aggregation. By judicious use of EPA and linoelic acid we can help optimize blood coagulation and other factors. I say "help optimize" because optimum health involves a cluster of interrelated factors, including diet, exercise, and supplements; emphasizing only one will not do.

Soon we may no longer have to consider osteoporosis as an inherent part of old age. The time may not be far off when bone density will be monitored like cholesterol and little old ladies with their frail bones will be part of nutrition history like goiters and cretinism. Optimizing bone density to prevent osteoporosis certainly requires balancing calcium, protein, and exercise. Again, supplementation is important, but so are diet and exercise.

In the near future, scientists will have a more thorough understanding of how nutrients can help us minimize the risk of cancer so that instead of three out of four families experiencing that tragedy, cancer will be a rare disease from the past like rickets or scurvy.

Perhaps, too, we will understand the oil called DHA and the role it plays in brain development so that we may benefit from that potential.

A mentor of mine used to say, "When you develop a new tool, apply it to an old problem." The old problem, as these pages tell, is to optimize nutrition by the effective use of supplementation. Our ancestors did this with the crude tools available to them by trial and error. We have tools that would seem like magic to them. To the extent that we apply these tools to the ongoing quest for optimum health, we and our children can enjoy to the fullest the greatest gift of each of us has: life.

Baseball great Satchel Paige once said it very well: "If I knew I would need this body so long, I would have taken better care of it much sooner." The means for taking better care of your body than humans have ever been able to do before are now at hand.

APPENDIX

Recommended Dietary Allowances (daily)

	Age (years)	Weight (kg)	Weight (lb)	Height (cm)	Height (in)	Protein (g)	Fat-Soluble Vitamins Vitamin A (μg RE)[a]	Fat-Soluble Vitamins Vitamin D (μg)[b]	Fat-Soluble Vitamins Vitamin E (mg α-TE)[c]
Infants	0.0–0.5	6	13	60	24	kg × 2.2	420	10	3
	0.5–1.0	9	20	71	28	kg × 2.0	400	10	4
Children	1–3	13	29	90	35	23	400	10	5
	4–6	20	44	112	44	30	500	10	6
	7–10	28	62	132	52	34	700	10	7
Males	11–14	45	99	157	62	45	1000	10	8
	15–18	66	145	176	69	56	1000	10	10
	19–22	70	154	177	70	56	1000	7.5	10
	23–50	70	154	178	70	56	1000	5	10
	51+	70	154	178	70	56	1000	5	10
Females	11–14	46	101	157	62	46	800	10	8
	15–18	55	120	163	64	46	800	10	8
	19–22	55	120	163	64	44	800	7.5	8
	23–50	55	120	163	64	44	800	5	8
	51+	55	120	163	64	44	800	5	8
Pregnant						+30	+200	+5	+2
Lactating						+20	+400	+5	+3

NOTE: The daily allowances are intended to provide for individual variations among most normal persons as they live in the United States under usual environmental stresses. Diets should be based on a variety of common foods in order to provide other nutrients for which human requirements have been less well defined.

[a] Retinol equivalents. 1 retinol equivalent = 1 μg retinol or 6 μg β carotene.

[b] As cholecalciferol. 10 μg cholecalciferol = 400 IU of vitamin D.

[c] α-tocopherol equivalents. 1 mg d-α tocopherol = 1 α-TE.

[d] 1 NE (niacin equivalent) is equal to 1 mg of niacin or 60 mg of dietary tryptophan.

[e] The folacin allowances refer to dietary sources as determined by *Lactobacillus casei* assay after treatment with enzymes (conjugases) to make polyglutamyl forms of the vitamin available to the test organism.

Water-Soluble Vitamins							Minerals					
Vitamin C (mg)	Thiamin (mg)	Riboflavin (mg)	Niacin (mg NE)^d	Vitamin B-6 (mg)	Folacin^e (μg)	Vitamin B-12 (μg)	Calcium (mg)	Phosphorus (mg)	Magnesium (mg)	Iron (mg)	Zinc (mg)	Iodine (μg)
35	0.3	0.4	6	0.3	30	0.5^f	360	240	50	10	3	40
35	0.5	0.6	8	0.6	45	1.5	540	360	70	15	5	50
45	0.7	0.8	9	0.9	100	2.0	800	800	150	15	10	70
45	0.9	1.0	11	1.3	200	2.5	800	800	200	10	10	90
45	1.2	1.4	16	1.6	300	3.0	800	800	250	10	10	120
50	1.4	1.6	18	1.8	400	3.0	1200	1200	350	18	15	150
60	1.4	1.7	18	2.0	400	3.0	1200	1200	400	18	15	150
60	1.5	1.7	19	2.2	400	3.0	800	800	350	10	15	150
60	1.4	1.6	18	2.2	400	3.0	800	800	350	10	15	150
60	1.2	1.4	16	2.2	400	3.0	800	800	350	10	15	150
50	1.1	1.3	15	1.8	400	3.0	1200	1200	300	18	15	150
60	1.1	1.3	14	2.0	400	3.0	1200	1200	300	18	15	150
60	1.1	1.3	14	2.0	400	3.0	800	800	300	18	15	150
60	1.0	1.2	13	2.0	400	3.0	800	800	300	18	15	150
60	1.0	1.2	13	2.0	400	3.0	800	800	300	10	15	150
+20	+0.4	+0.3	+2	+0.6	+400	+1.0	+400	+400	+150	g	+5	+25
+40	+0.5	+0.5	+5	+0.5	+100	+1.0	+400	+400	+150	g	+10	+50

^{f}The recommended dietary allowance for vitamin B-12 in infants is based on average concentration of the vitamin in human milk. The allowances after weaning are based on energy intake (as recommended by the American Academy of Pediatrics) and consideration of other factors, such as intestinal absorption.

^{g}The increased requirement during pregnancy cannot be met by the iron content of habitual American diets nor by the existing iron stores of many women; therefore the use of 30–60 mg of supplemental iron is recommended. Iron needs during lactation are not substantially different from those of nonpregnant women, but continued supplementation of the mother for 2–3 months after parturition is advisable in order to replenish stores depleted by pregnancy.

SOURCE: Adapted from *Recommended Dietary Allowances*, 9th revised edition, 1980, with permission of the National Academy of Sciences, Washington.

SUGGESTED READING

This reading list is by no means comprehensive. It will provide the interested reader with sources readily available in any good library for more detailed investigation. Some of the readings refer to specific materials mentioned in this book.

General

Briggs, George B., and Doris Howes Calloway. *Nutrition and Physical Fitness.* 11th ed. New York: Holt, Rinehart and Winston, 1984.

Deutsch, Ronald M. *Realities of Nutrition.* Palo Alto: Bull, 1976.

Farb, Peter, and George Armelugos. *Consuming Passions: The Anthropology of Eating.* Boston: Houghton Mifflin, 1980.

Hooker, Richard J. *Food and Drink in America.* Indianapolis/New York: Bobbs-Merrill, 1981.

Nunnelley, Eva May, and Eleanor Noss Whitney. *Concepts and Controversies in Nutrition.* 2d ed. St. Paul, Minn.: West, 1982.

Whitney, Eleanor Noss, and Eva May Nunnelley Hamilton. *Understanding Nutrition.* 3d ed. St. Paul, Minn.: West, 1984.

Chapter 1: Dietary Fiber

Burkitt, Denis. *Eat Right to Stay Healthy and Enjoy Life More: How Simple Diet Changes Can Prevent Many Common Diseases.* New York: Arco, 1979.

Spiller, Gene A., and H. J. Freeman. "Dietary Fiber in Human Nutrition." In J. Weininger and G. M. Briggs, eds., *Nutrition Update*. Vol. 1. New York: John Wiley, 1983.

Story, Jon A., and D. Kritchevsky. "Nutrients with Special Functions: Dietary Fiber." In R. B. Alfin-Slater and D. Kritchevsky, eds., *Human Nutrition: A Comprehensive Treatise*. New York: Plenum, 1980.

Chapter 2: Vitamin A

Freeman, Hugh James. "Retinoids and Carcinogenesis." In Gene Spiller, ed., *Current Topics in Nutrition and Disease*. Vol. 4: *Nutritional Pharmacology*. New York: Alan R. Liss, 1981.

Michaëlson, G., et al. "Effects of Oral Zinc and Vitamin A in Acne." *Archives of Dermatology* 113 (1977): 31–36.

Peto, R., et al. "Can Dietary Beta-Carotene Materially Reduce Human Cancer Rates?" *Nature* 290 (1981): 201–8.

Shekelle, R. B., et al. "Dietary Vitamin A and the Risk of Cancer in the Western Electric Study." *Lancet* (1981): 1185–90.

Chapter 3: Vitamin D

General readings apply (see page 196).

Chapter 4: Vitamins E and K

Haeger, K., et al. "Long-time Treatment of Intermittent Claudication with Vitamin E." *American Journal of Clinical Nutrition* 27 (1974); 1179.

Natta, C., et al. "Plasma Levels of Tocopherol in Sickle Cell Anemia Subjects." *American Journal of Clinical Nutrition* 32 (1979): 1359–62.

Tappel, A. L., et al. "Effects of Exercise, Vitamin E, and Ozone on Pulmonary Function and Lipid Peroxidation." *Journal of Applied Physiology* 45 (1978): 927–32.

Vitamin E: A Comprehensive Treatise. In Lawrence J. Machlin, ed. New York: Marcel Dekker, 1980.

Chapter 5: Vitamin C

Basu, T. K., and C. J. Solbrar. *Vitamin C in Health and Disease.* Westport, Conn.: AVI, 1982.

Eaton, S. Boyd, and Melvin Konner. "Paleolithic Nutrition: A Consideration of Its Nature and Current Implications." *New England Journal of Medicine* 312 (1985): 283–89.

Hughes, R. E. *Vitamin C: Some Current Problems.* London: British Nutrition Foundation, 1981.

Chapter 6: The B Vitamins

Editors of Consumer Guide. *The Vitamin Book.* New York: Simon and Schuster, 1979.

Whitney, Eleanor Noss, and Eva May Nunnelley Hamilton. *Understanding Nutrition.* 3d ed. St. Paul, Minn.: West, 1984.

Chapter 7: Calcium

Albanese, Anthony A. *Current Topics in Nutrition and Disease.* Vol. 1: *Bone Loss: Causes, Detection and Therapy.* New York: Alan R. Liss, 1977.

McCarron, David, et al. "The Calcium–Blood Pressure Hypothesis: Evidence for Its Validity." *Contemporary Nutrition* 9 (1984): no. 11.

Notelovitz, Morris, and Marsha Ware. *Stand Tall: The Informed Woman's Guide to Preventing Osteoporosis.* Gainesville, Fla.: Triad, 1982.

Chapter 8: Iron

Food and Nutrition Board. *Trace Elements in Human and Animal Nutrition.* 4th ed. New York: Academic, 1980.

Chapter 9: Trace Minerals

Eby, George A., et al. "Reduction in Duration of Common Colds by Zinc Gluconate Lozenges in a Double-Blind Study." *Antimicrobial Agents and Chemotherapy* 25 (1984): 20–24.

Underwood, Eric J. *Trace Elements in Human and Animal Nutrition.* 4th ed. New York: Academic, 1977.

Chapter 10: Pregnancy

Hess, Mary Abbott, and Anne Elise. *Pickles and Ice Cream: The Complete Guide to Nutrition During Pregnancy.* New York: Dell, 1984.

Chapter 11: Electrolytes

Eaton, S. Boyd. "Paleolithic Nutrition: A Consideration of Its Nature and Current Implications." *New England Journal of Medicine* 312 (1985): 283–89.

Margie, Joyce D., and James C. Hunt. *Living with High Blood Pressure: The Hypertension Diet Cookbook.* Edited by Robert Offergeld. Bloomfield, Ill.: HLS Press, 1978.

Netzer, Corinne. *The Low-Salt Diet Encounter.* New York: Dell, 1982.

Chapter 12: EPA

Chaintreuil, J., et al. "Effects of Dietary Gamma-Linolenate Supplementation on Serum Lipids and Platelet Function in Insulin-Dependent Diabetic Patients." *Human Nutrition and Clinical Nutrition* 38 (1984): 121–30.

Goodnight, S. H., Jr.; W. S. Harris; W. E. Connor; and D. Roger Illingworth: "Polyunsaturated Fatty Acids, Hyperlipidemia, and Thrombosis." *Arteriosclerosis* 2 (March/April 1982): 87–113.

Horrobin, D. F. "The Role of Essential Fatty Acids and Prostaglandins in the Premenstrual Syndrome." *Journal of Reproductive Medicine* 28 (1983): 405–8.

Pigott, George M. *The Pathway to a Healthy Heart.* Seal Beach, Cal.: Scientific Nutrition Press, 1983.

Chapter 13: Diet and Cancer

Cancer Prevention, February 1984, No. 84-2671. Bethesda, Md.: NIH.

Committee on Diet, Nutrition, and Cancer. *Diet, Nutrition and Cancer.* Washington: National Academy Press, 1982.

DiSogra, Charles, and Lorelei Groll. *Diet, Nutrition and Cancer Prevention: A Guide to Food Choices.* Bethesda, Md.: National Cancer Institute.

Rainer, R., et al. "Reduction of Gastric Carcinogenesis with Ascorbic

Acid." *New York Academy of Science: Annals* 258 (1975): 181–89.

Spiller, Gene A., and Ruth McPherson Kay, eds. *Medical Aspects of Dietary Fiber.* New York: Plenum, 1980.

Wassertheil-Smoller, S., et al. "Dietary Vitamin C and Uterine Cervical Dysplasia." *American Journal of Epidemiology* 114 (1981): 714–24.

Chapter 14: How All This Came to Pass

Library of Health. *Wholesome Diet.* Alexandria, Va.: Time-Life Books, 1981.

Science and Education Administration/Human Nutrition, U.S. Department of Agriculture. *Ideas for Better Eating: Menus and Recipes to Make Use of the Dietary Guidelines.* Washington: U.S. Government Printing Office, 1981.

———. *Food: The Hassle-Free Guide to a Better Diet.* Washington: U.S. Government Printing Office, 1979.

Wurtman, Judith A. *Eating Your Way Through Life: A No-Nonsense Guide to Good Nutrition for All Ages and All Eating Styles.* New York: Raven Press, 1979.

INDEX

About the Author

JAMES SCALA devotes his life to making sound nutritional information accessible to the average person. He has been involved in nutrition and health research for over twenty years.

After completing undergraduate work at Columbia, Dr. Scala received his Ph.D. in biochemistry from Cornell University in 1964. He has taught nutrition at various universities and medical schools in the United States and abroad. He has published many articles on food nutrition and health.

Most of all, though, he enjoys talking about nutrition to the general public. His ability to discuss complex nutrition-related health issues in an accurate and understandable way makes him a frequent guest on radio and television talk shows.

Dr. Scala is vice-president of Science and Technology for the Shaklee Corporation. His experience in nutrition science and the business world gives him a unique insight into the basics of nutrition and the impact of societal trends on the way people eat.

An avid sailor and astronomer, Dr. Scala lives near San Francisco with his wife and children.